Not Your Grandmother's Nursing Home

Not

Your Grandmother's Nursing Home

Demystifying Today's Retirement Living Options

Elizabeth L. Bewley

ISBN:1490302417
ISBN-13:9781490302416

DEDICATION

For everyone who is now—or one day will be—
trying to make sense of retirement living options

CONTENTS

ACKNOWLEDGMENTS

Thanks go to my editor Tim Wiederaenders at the Prescott, AZ *Daily Courier.* Without his support, my weekly newspaper column "The Good Patient" would not exist, and neither would this book.

I appreciate the willingness of people interviewed to offer information and insight. I am glad for the engagement of readers, whose questions and comments highlighted topics that needed additional explanation.

I remain perpetually grateful to my husband, Stephen R. Brubaker, whose roles include thoughtful audience and devil's advocate, photographer, and book designer.

INTRODUCTION

I decided to write two or three articles about retirement living options for my column, "The Good Patient," in the Prescott, AZ *Daily Courier.* I planned to explain the differences among independent living, assisted living, and skilled nursing.

The planned articles expanded to become forty columns.

Responses to my efforts to explain a complex topic have been very positive. A number of readers asked that I publish the columns in a book, which you now have before you.

Please check with any individual retirement communities you are considering before making any decisions based on information herein, for at least two reasons.

First, information can change over time. Second, the communities often are able to offer customized options and alternatives. It never hurts to ask.

I

Retirement Communities Defined

For the first set of articles, I researched, visited and conducted many interviews at retirement communities run by four organizations across five campuses in the Prescott, AZ area. (Good Samaritan operates in two locations; sometimes for simplicity's sake I refer to these as one.)

I chose communities that offer independent living as well as assisted living. Most also offer skilled nursing and/or memory care (dementia care).

These sites are not the only options in the area, but they offer the broadest range of services under one umbrella.

If you are interested in communities elsewhere, these articles can help you understand a representative range of options, to aid you in deciding what questions you want to ask of any retirement community you consider.

1

Retirement Communities: Not Your Grandmother's Nursing Home

When I was 10 years old, I went Christmas caroling with a church group to a nursing home. The whole place seemed to be done up in various shades of brown—a sepia-toned photograph brought to life.

As I recall, the floor was covered in linoleum, worn through in places. The halls were dark and dank and smelled funny. The rooms were tiny and drab. The very building seemed dispirited. We sang our songs and left.

I went home and had nightmares.

If you have similar memories from many decades ago, I have good news for you. The retirement communities I've toured in Prescott are as different from the place I remember from childhood as dining at a five-

3

star restaurant is different from scavenging for food in a dumpster.

Yes, both eating experiences have to do with getting food—and both sets of retirement experiences have to do with having a place to live—but the similarities end there.

What can you expect from today's senior living communities?

My comments here are based on tours of Alta Vista, Good Samaritan, Granite Gate, and Las Fuentes.

For one thing, the basics appear to be well covered. Three of the four are affiliates of national organizations that run retirement communities in as many as hundreds of locations across the U.S. (Alta Vista, on the other hand, is locally owned.)

They all understand very clearly that you want to have a pleasant, clean and safe place to live. You'd like choices for meals. You need a way to get laundry done.

You need to get to a grocery store, a drug store, the post office and the doctor's office—even if you don't plan to drive yourself. You want to be able to get beauty salon or barber services without leaving the site.

You want interesting things to do—and interesting people to do them with—even if you aren't up for organizing the activities or driving to get to them. You may want the ability to entertain guests even if you don't have space for them to stay with you.

You may want help with computers and internet access. Maybe you want to be able to Skype (make free video calls via computer) with your relatives even if you aren't sure how to set that service up.

Maybe you want to know that someone will keep an eye on you—not an intrusive eye, if you are living independently in your own apartment—but just that someone will notice if you don't surface one day.

Above all, you want to be treated as the individual you are—if you need something different from the service offerings already available, you want to know that you'll be taken seriously and that management will help you get what you need.

In all the communities, the staff made a convincing case that they have these bases covered.

In all the communities, staff and residents uniformly greeted each other warmly in the hallways—and the staff almost always knew the name of every single resident we happened upon.

It sometimes took a while to make our way down a hall—it was common for residents to stop staff members to share some point of interest about their activities or their families. And the staff always knew the backstory—what had happened previously with the resident's family member or vacation plans or whatever.

Retirement organizations like these make a point of referring to themselves as "communities" rather than as "facilities" or "developments" or anything else.

At first, I thought that this emphasis was simply a marketing ploy. But after spending many hours on these campuses, I'm convinced that they're completely serious: they offer a chance to experience community.

Future columns will highlight some differences among the communities. But know that residents express satisfaction—and often delight—in all four. One resident of Las Fuentes concluded, in a fast-moving conversation with half a dozen residents, "I can't believe that in my old age, I'm having more fun than I've had my whole life!"

2

Independent Living:
What Is It?

The house is getting to be too much to take care of, cooking seems like a chore, and you really, really don't want to be climbing ladders to change light bulbs any more. If you consider moving to something called a "retirement community," what exactly does that mean?

As used in this column, a retirement community is a campus that offers not only independent living arrangements—typically apartments—but also assisted living arrangements and possibly facilities that provide additional levels of care such as a skilled nursing unit.

They set a minimum age for residents, typically 55 or 62, but if one spouse meets the age limit and the other doesn't, they can generally work around that requirement.

What does independent living mean? As in non-retirement apartment complexes, you retain complete control over your schedule and your activities. (Well, okay, loud parties at 4 a.m. are frowned upon, no matter where you live.)

Small well-behaved pets with valid licenses are typically welcome. If you want to bring your car, that's fine, too.

What is an independent living apartment like? The four sites visited for this column—Alta Vista, Good Samaritan, Granite Gate, and Las Fuentes—offer dozens of different floor plans ranging from studios that are less than 500 square feet to a penthouse of more than 1700 square feet.

Most common, though, are one- and two-bedroom apartments of roughly 600-1000 square feet. Good Samaritan also offers casitas (900-1400 square feet).

Each site requires a one-time fee that you pay before you move in, but these are not the massive buy-in fees that you may be familiar with from other parts of the country. They range from $50-$300 at Good Samaritan to $2500 at Alta Vista.

Good Samaritan in Prescott does have an option for its casitas of a largely refundable entrance fee coupled with smaller monthly payments, but there is no requirement that new residents choose this approach.

Apartments are unfurnished, but are outfitted with standard kitchen appliances—stove, refrigerator, etc.—and with a washer and dryer if the apartment is designed with space for them.

When an apartment becomes available, it is typical for the carpet to be replaced and for the unit to be completely repainted. If you want colors other than the standard ones offered, Las Fuentes will even offer to paint your apartment whatever color you like—as long as you provide the paint.

The apartments in the different communities offer different appealing features. For example, at Granite Gate, each apartment has a striking view of the rocks of Granite Dells. At Good Samaritan in Prescott Valley, the apartments have bay windows.

At Las Fuentes, the apartments tend to be larger, and most have walk-in pantries. In Alta Vista, apartment kitchens have granite counters and hardwood cherry cabinets.

Options for meals vary. At Alta Vista, no meals are included in the base rate, but they offer three meals a day in various upscale settings. Meals can be purchased one at a time, and monthly packages are also available. At Granite Gate, the base rate—even for independent living— includes three meals a day.

Good Samaritan in Prescott Valley includes a mid-day meal 20 days a month in its base rate—and has no objection if residents bring storage containers with them at lunch, and take home some extra soup and/or salad for dinner. At Good Samaritan in Prescott, all meals are optional.

Las Fuentes offers three restaurant-style meals a day, and a variety of meal plans. Because it sells packages of meal tickets, residents typically don't lose money if they skip meals, even if they have signed up for a package plan, because the meal tickets do not expire.

Three important points to take away are: first, the apartment options for independent living in retirement communities are quite varied and each offers a different appeal.

Second, meal plans are often very flexible.

Third, if you've assumed that you wouldn't like any retirement community apartments or meal arrangements, you might be pleasantly surprised at the options available to you.

3

Independent Living:
The Experience

What is independent living like in a retirement community? In a word, busy—if you want it to be.

You may spend more time at meals than you have before, because you may enjoy talking with new friends. And you just might find the meals more appealing than the cheese sandwiches you'd been eating by default at home.

At Good Samaritan in Prescott Valley, you may linger to enjoy live piano music often played by volunteers during lunch. Las Fuentes offers live music at its popular Thursday lunchtime buffet, and at Saturday dinner.

Sample recent menu items for independent living residents at some of the retirement communities in town follow.

11

- Granite Gate: marinated steak on garden salad; roast pork loin
- Good Samaritan in Prescott Valley: chicken cordon bleu; beef and broccoli stir-fry
- Alta Vista: filet mignon wrapped in bacon; chicken Parmesan with gluten-free pasta
- Las Fuentes: lobster Newburg; chicken Wellington

The sites offer a wide variety of activities, both onsite and offsite. All offer transportation services, and have their own buses to take people on outings to casinos, ballgames, golf, swimming, parks, and community cultural events such as concerts on the town square.

Music, gardening, movies, travelogues, art, Bible study and other religious and spiritual activities, crafts, yoga, stretching or other health activities, book groups, jigsaw puzzles, Wii fitness games, bingo, and other games are offered in most of the communities. A few activities reported at specific communities are noted here.

- Good Samaritan: poker, pet therapy with visiting dogs, monthly birthday parties
- Las Fuentes: trips to dinner theatre in Phoenix; outings to new restaurants; a Write Your Life class
- Alta Vista: onsite Corvette car show; cooking demos; Granite Creek vineyards outing
- Granite Gate: Rummikub (a game that reportedly "combines elements of rummy, dominoes, mah-jongg and chess"); Lynx Lake outing; men's group

Support services for people in independent living are surprisingly extensive. For example, all four organizations offer transportation at no extra charge for doctors' appointments and shopping.

All four keep an eye out to make sure that people surface at least once a day. For example, at Las Fuentes, residents must press a button to turn off a blinking light on a call system in the bathroom by 10 a.m., or the staff will check on them.

Since three meals a day are included in the basic package at Granite Gate, if a resident doesn't show up for a meal, the staff will go look for them.

Further, Granite Gate residents are all encouraged to wear emergency call pendants—and the staff monitors battery life, and replaces batteries before they fail.

If you plan to be away for the day, or out of town for a while—or even just prefer to sleep until noon—it is a simple matter to let the staff know not to come looking for you until you expect to be available.

The most surprising fact about the arrangements in all of the communities is how flexible they are and how willing the staff is to try to meet your needs if you want— or are interested in—something that's not standard.

At Alta Vista, one of the residents has a granddaughter who is a kindergarten teacher. When the kindergarten puts on a show, Alta Vista provides a sign-up sheet and a bus, and a bus full of residents goes to see the five-year-olds perform.

At Las Fuentes, staff from the physical therapy department goes to the fitness center once a week and will work with any resident on anything they want, at no charge.

If people are in the hospital, staff from Resident Services will visit them, water their plants, pick up their mail, and take care of other things residents may need until they come home.

At Granite Gate, a Residents' Council tells management what they want—such as benches and picnic tables—and management makes changes accordingly.

At Good Samaritan in Prescott, a rotating display gives residents a chance to showcase their hobbies, interests, and expertise for other residents.

4

Assisted Living:
What Is It?

Your spouse requires help bathing and dressing, and it is getting to be too much for you to manage his or her pill regimen. Sometimes you look in the cupboard and you're reminded of an old TV show in which a woman is trying to prepare a meal with the only two ingredients on hand—spaghetti noodles and chocolate sauce.

Your children have suggested assisted living. But what exactly is that?

AARP says, "Assisted living residences are aimed at helping residents remain as self-sufficient as possible with the assurance of assistance when needed. A combination of housing, meals, personal care and support, social activities, 24-hour supervision and, in some residences, health-related services is usually provided."

Assisted living generally implies living in an apartment very much like an independent living apartment, although typically with a microwave in the kitchen rather than a full stove and oven.

Assisted living is sometimes viewed as one type of long-term care.

In Arizona, assisted living centers have to follow a large number of very specific rules. They must provide three nutritious meals a day and a snack—and dinner and breakfast cannot be more than 14 hours apart. Menus must be dated and posted at least a week ahead of time.

The facility has to ensure that "daily social, recreational, or rehabilitative activities are provided" that meet "residents' preferences, needs, and abilities." A calendar of activities must be posted at least a week in advance.

Residents must be provided "encouragement and assistance to preserve outside support systems" and "social interaction to maintain identity and self-worth."

The site must provide daily newspapers, current magazines "and a variety of reading materials." These are typically made available in common areas, often onsite libraries.

The site must offer a "hazard-free outdoor area with shaded protection where residents may walk or sit." Interestingly, the facility must be free of odors.

Assisted living sites must "conspicuously post" residents' rights, and provide residents with information about how to resolve grievances.

The sites are required to keep on file the name and contact information for a family member or other representative who can be notified if any problems arise and who can make decisions on behalf of the resident if necessary.

The regulations spell out three different levels of care, and a site may not accept as a resident someone who requires a higher level of care than it is licensed to provide.

The three levels of care are as follows.

The first level is "supervisory care," which means that residents are able to handle without assistance basic activities like bathing, dressing, and eating meals provided, and also need very little help managing any medicines.

The second level is "personal care," which means that they may need some nursing services, have one or more medical conditions that require monitoring, need help managing medicines, and need assistance with one or more activities such as bathing, dressing, and walking.

The third level is "directed care," which means that the individual is "incapable of recognizing danger, summoning assistance, expressing need or making basic care decisions." Residents may need extensive help with bathing, dressing, getting to meals, and so forth. They need to be monitored frequently because of physical or cognitive limitations.

Of the four communities visited for this series, Good Samaritan, Las Fuentes, and Granite Gate all offer all three levels of care; Alta Vista offers the first two but not the third.

When people move into an assisted living facility, a service plan must be prepared within fourteen days.

It is developed with input from the resident and/or the resident's representative, and specifies the level of assisted living service and any medical services that the individual will be receiving. It is signed by the resident/representative and by site staff.

The law provides many protections; it is still important to be attentive in choosing a site.

AARP offers a checklist that identifies a wide range of topics to cover when considering assisted living sites at http://assets.aarp.org/external_sites/caregiving/checklists/checklist_assistedLiving.html.

The Arizona Department of Health Services offers its own explanation of assisted living and a checklist at http://www.azdhs.gov/als/guides/achbro.pdf.

See licensing information and inspection reports at http://hsapps.azdhs.gov/ls/sod/SearchProv.aspx?type=AL. (Good Samaritan's site in Prescott is listed under the unit's name, which is Willow Wind.)

5

Assisted Living:
The Experience

Here is a little quiz for you. Identify in what living arrangements locally you will find:

1. A large vegetable garden in an interior courtyard, which provides enough eggplant for the chef to make eggplant parmesan for everyone, and enough fruit to permit home-made jam to be served at breakfast

2. A once-a-week "spa" experience with a relaxing hour in a jetted tub, followed by a massage and a pedicure, at no extra charge

3. A continuous loop hallway, so that people who might have trouble finding their living quarters know that if they just keep walking, they will eventually reach home

4. Three large, interior courtyards, so that people who easily get lost have several completely safe places to go outside and enjoy the fine weather, on their own

5. All meals served restaurant style, available over a 2-1/2 hour span for each meal, so that people can eat when they like

6. Elegant nameplates for each door, in hallways that look like a lovely hotel

7. Help surfing the internet and/or staying in touch with families via email or Skype, even if you are fuzzy about how computers work

8. Full access to all activities offered to any group in the retirement community

9. No need to move from the apartment you have been living in independently even if you start to need assisted living services, because all services are delivered to people who need them regardless of their location

10. Uniformly stunning views, no matter what type of apartment you live in

11. Apartments that range from more than 500 square feet to almost 1400 square feet

12. No complications if one person in a couple needs assisted living and the other does not, with no need for one person to move to another apartment on the campus, because it is part of the standard offering that tailored services are delivered wherever they are needed

13. The option to eat in any of several dining venues, routinely enjoying meals such as eggs benedict, seafood primavera on gluten-free pasta, and fresh Atlantic salmon—your choice of grilled, poached, or seared

14. The chance to take part in cooking demonstrations with the chef, in a well-equipped test kitchen

15. Upscale interiors, starting with a sweeping spiral staircase in the lobby

16. Free transportation not just for shopping and doctors' appointments, but for other personal appointments as well

The answer: all of these are features of assisted living arrangements in retirement communities in Prescott. (Items 1-4 are found at Good Samaritan; 5-8 at Las Fuentes; 9-12 at Granite Gate; and 13-16 at Alta Vista.)

When I first planned to check out the assisted living arrangements in these communities, I prepared a spreadsheet with nearly a hundred questions:

How long has the site been operating? How many square feet are the apartments? What do the apartments cost? What are the charges for different levels of additional care? Is there staff onsite 24/7? How many people live there?

I have gathered much of the information, and it is useful to have. However, I feel a bit like the aviator in *The Little Prince*. He is fussing over quantifiable facts concerning his airplane, which has suffered mechanical failure in the middle of a desert. The little prince, who has inexplicably arrived from a distant asteroid, is concerned with matters of the heart.

The aviator later explains this distinction, saying, "Grown-ups love figures. When you tell them that you have made a new friend, they never ask you any questions about essential matters. They never say to you, 'What does his voice sound like? What games does he love best? Does he collect butterflies?' Instead, they demand, 'How old is he? How many brothers has he? How much does he weigh? How much money does his father make?' Only from these figures do they think they have learned anything about him."

The "essential matters" concerning retirement communities may have less to do with square feet and more to do with the heart of each place. While I will touch on this point in future columns, you may want to go see for yourself.

6

Nursing/Skilled Nursing: What Is It?

The federal government makes a distinction between "skilled nursing facilities" whose residents require extensive medical care, and "nursing facilities," which provide care that is more custodial in nature.

The second of these is what most people think of as nursing homes. These are also often referred to as long-term care facilities.

Of the four retirement communities visited for this series, Good Samaritan and Las Fuentes offer nursing/skilled nursing. Granite Gate and Alta Vista do not.

The facilities at Good Samaritan and Las Fuentes carry dual certification, which means that they are licensed as both "skilled nursing" and "nursing" facilities.

Both organizations offer short-term rehabilitation and long-term care.

Short-term rehab centers typically house individuals for just a few weeks, often as they recover from surgery such as a knee or hip replacement. Rehab centers also offer outpatient services.

Long-term care facilities are home to people who—because of physical or cognitive impairment—are unable to take care of themselves, require care 24/7, and typically are expected to stay in that setting as long as they live.

Both Good Samaritan and Las Fuentes separate short-term rehab and long-term care populations, housing them in different corridors.

The people in rehab tend to be about 15 years younger than those in long-term care. They typically spend hours each day in physical and occupational therapy. The units house one or two people per room.

The facilities are licensed under a combination of federal and state regulations. Many core requirements for sites that want to be eligible for any federal funding from Medicare are spelled out in federal rules. These have many elements similar to state rules for a lower level of care, assisted living.

For example, the facilities must arrange "an ongoing program of activities designed to meet. . . the interests and the physical, mental, and psychosocial well-being of each resident."

Such programs variously need to "provide stimulation or solace; promote physical, cognitive, and/or emotional health; enhance, to the extent practicable, each resident's physical and mental status; and promote each resident's self-respect by providing, for example, activities that support self-expression and choice."

Guidelines for inspectors ask, "Are residents who are confined or choose to remain in their rooms provided with in room activities in keeping with life-long interests (e.g., music, reading, visits with individuals who share their interests or reasonable attempts to connect the resident with such individuals) and in-room projects they can work on independently? Do any facility staff members assist the resident with activities he or she can pursue independently?"

The facilities are also required to arrange for medically-related social services. These include, for example, "making referrals and obtaining services from outside entities (e.g., talking books, absentee ballots)" and "assisting residents with financial and legal matters (e.g., applying for pensions, referrals to lawyers.)"

Facilities are also advised that they must address needs for a "home-like environment, control, dignity, and privacy."

For example, facilities are expected to encourage residents to bring as many personal possessions as they want, including furniture, that can safely be accommodated in their rooms (or their half of a room.)

The Arizona Department of Health Services offers information about and guidance for choosing a nursing home at http://www.azdhs.gov/als/ltc/nhconsgde.pdf.

Medicare offers a comprehensive nursing home checklist at http://www.medicare.gov/files/nursing-home-checklist.pdf.

States are charged with inspecting nursing/skilled nursing facilities and deciding whether they meet Medicare's requirements.

See the results of Arizona state inspections on the Arizona Department of Health Services website at http://hsapps.azdhs.gov/ls/sod/SearchProv.aspx?type=LTC.

One piece of good news that you will be able to see is that neither Las Fuentes nor Good Samaritan has been the subject of any enforcement actions for the three years whose inspection results the site posts.

The federal government also offers information at http://www.medicare.gov/NursingHomeCompare.

That site allows you to look up information about any nursing home, and to compare nursing homes on a wide variety of measures—for example, what percentage of long-term care residents have had falls that result in serious injuries.

Online comparisons, though, do not do away with the need to visit in person to get a feel for the place.

7

Nursing/Skilled Nursing:
The Experience

This article focuses on nursing/skilled nursing facilities that provide long-term care in two retirement communities, Good Samaritan and Las Fuentes. (The other two communities visited for this series, Alta Vista and Granite Gate, do not offer these units.)

One remarkable fact about these facilities, compared to others with which I am familiar, is how quiet they are.

Every facility has patient alarm systems. Some alarms are triggered when residents press a call button.

Others are triggered when people with some cognitive limitations try to do something that is unsafe for them. For example, if it is unsafe for someone to get out of bed unaided, his bed may be fitted with a pressure pad that sends an alarm if he is no longer lying down.

In many facilities, it is not unusual to hear alarms go off every few minutes. At the sites I visited, I did not hear any.

Residents generally seemed to be quietly occupied, either in their rooms or in group activities. Pet therapy dogs are common sights in the long-term care units. Most residents eat in the dining rooms.

Good Samaritan provides unusual training to new administrators (top executives) of its nursing/skilled nursing facilities.

They are picked up by a van at home, transported in a wheelchair, taken to live in the nursing/skilled nursing facility for two or three days, and treated like every other resident. They develop a profound understanding of what it is like to have to depend on others.

At Good Samaritan, volunteers routinely play the piano for residents at lunch. Unexpected upgrades, such as leather couches in various nooks, are common.

These were often bought with money donated to this nonprofit organization for that purpose by families who appreciate the care given to their relatives.

You might be surprised at how engaged long-term care residents are. Good Samaritan employees help them with email, internet access, and Skyping with their families.

An activities staff offers many outings, including ones to Tim's Toyota Center, a venue that seats 5000-plus people for sporting and cultural events.

Good Samaritan is working to upgrade its facilities in several ways. Vacated rooms in Prescott Valley are renovated with wood flooring, dark wood armoires, and flat screen TVs. A new Electronic Medical Records system, or EMR, is expected to be up and running in March 2013. EMRs promise increased efficiency, safety, and accuracy in tracking patient status, care, and needs.

Las Fuentes offers the largest nursing/skilled nursing unit (128 beds). Its size allows it to have a doctor onsite four days a week—an unusual and reassuring feature.

It has a beauty salon right in the unit, and a dedicated ice cream parlor where free ice cream socials are hosted three days a week. It allows smoking (on an outside patio, under supervision.)

It offers a wide variety of activities, including games such as bingo and blackjack. Free manicures are offered weekly.

The Las Fuentes physical plant has some limitations. The only central gathering place is a windowless dining room. Some residents were observed simply sitting in wheelchairs in the hallways. Furniture and carpeting in some rooms I glanced into seemed quite a bit worse for the wear.

That said, the Las Fuentes staff showed a genuine, heartfelt commitment to their residents, and showed creativity in meeting their needs.

If a facility has only one bed available and is faced with two potential residents who have equal needs, one who resides in their retirement community and one who does not, they are likely to give priority to the one who already lives in their retirement community.

In practice, though, typically about half the residents in nursing/skilled nursing at both Las Fuentes and Good Samaritan have come from outside the retirement community itself—they had been living in their own houses or in apartments not affiliated with the facility. They may even have been living in a different retirement community.

Said another way, assuming that space is available, nothing stops assisted living residents at Alta Vista or Granite Gate from moving to Good Samaritan or Las Fuentes if they need long-term care.

8

Memory Care:
The Experience

Memory care facilities are intended for people who have Alzheimer's or another form of dementia or cognitive impairment and who are at risk because they tend to wander away from their living quarters without having the ability to find their way back or to ask for help.

These facilities typically have locked doors to help ensure that residents remain in the unit unless they are escorted out.

People with dementia who do not wander may often reside in standard assisted living units or nursing facilities.

Good Samaritan in Prescott Valley and Granite Gate in Prescott offer memory care facilities. Las Fuentes and Alta Vista do not.

Memory care at Granite Gate takes place in an assisted living unit. Residents live in appealing apartments that offer nearly 400 square feet of space and contain several large closets.

Rena Phillips, Executive Director of Granite Gate, commented, "I lived in one of these apartments when I first came here, before I found another place to stay."

Outside each apartment is a large clear acrylic box mounted on the wall at eye level. Each contains a tastefully arranged collection of pictures, text, and mementos that help residents both remember who they are and quickly tell which room is theirs.

The Good Samaritan memory care unit, which it calls its Special Care Unit, is licensed as a nursing/skilled nursing facility. Resident rooms are typical of rooms in their other nursing/skilled nursing units, rather than apartments.

The trade-off is that Good Samaritan is able to offer a broader range of services than Granite Gate is licensed to provide.

Memory care units are quite pleasant at both Good Samaritan (16 residents) and Granite Gate (30 residents). An air of calm and quiet pervades both.

I have seen other skilled nursing facilities for people with dementia where one is constantly jarred by shouts and moans of residents, by alarms going off, and by loud instructions from staff members to residents who are unsteady on their feet, telling them to sit down when they try to stand up unaided.

I did not see or hear a single instance of any of those disruptions in either the Granite Gate or Good Samaritan memory care units.

The common areas in both facilities have ample space and lots of natural light. Public space at Good Samaritan feels cozy and homelike; Granite Gate offers a larger open area with soaring ceilings.

At both facilities I visited, most of the residents were out of their rooms and seated in the common areas. They were cheerfully engaged in various activities, with staff working to assist them. At both sites, staff members have been specially trained to work with people with dementia.

Under rules for both assisted living and nursing/skilled nursing, facilities are required to offer an extensive program of daily activities that meet the needs of their residents.

These rules apply just as much to units for people with dementia as they do to other units, and both sites appear to take this requirement seriously.

Granite Gate's memory care unit runs under a program called Bridge to Rediscovery.

It draws from Montessori principles. You may be familiar with Montessori as a teaching method used with children to help them be and feel successful. Some researchers have concluded that a similar approach can help people with dementia.

Good Samaritan has an activities staff in its memory care unit that works to create a wide variety of activities and outings. Contrary to popular belief, individuals in a memory care unit can leave the facility to enjoy experiences in the broader community, accompanied by aides who keep them safe.

Granite Gate runs a monthly support group for family members of its residents. This service can help people who are understandably troubled that parents or other relatives—who they remember as intelligent, passionate, driven, and successful—no longer remember basic facts about their lives and their families.

9

Moving From Independent Living To Assisted Living

Suppose that you move into an independent living apartment at Alta Vista, Good Samaritan, Granite Gate, or Las Fuentes and then over time it turns out that you need assisted living services. What arrangements are required to get that additional care?

The transition is easiest at Granite Gate: you stay in the apartment that you are already in. They bring the services to you.

This arrangement is especially useful when one spouse needs assisted living and the other one does not. And it is very convenient: no packing or unpacking is required, and there is no need to get used to being in a new space.

In the other communities, generally you would need to move to an apartment designated for assisted living, although there are exceptions.

Assisted living apartments are typically clustered in a separate wing with its own dining room/restaurant. Additional services are included. For example, snacks are available and residents are checked on several times a day.

If you were in independent living at Good Samaritan in Prescott Valley, to get assisted living services you would need to move to their assisted living unit in Prescott because they do not offer assisted living at their Prescott Valley campus.

At all of the sites except Granite Gate, for people to start getting assisted living services from the retirement community's organization, typically there has to be a vacancy in the assisted living wing.

But usually this constraint does not pose a problem. Because the need for assisted living services often develops gradually over time, residents or their representatives can generally work out this transition with the management of the retirement community.

What if you can't wait?

At Granite Gate, the issue simply doesn't arise, since no move is needed. At the other three communities, if the site's management can't arrange for services to come to the resident, then residents or their representatives can make arrangements on their own for outside agencies to send nurses and/or non-medical aides to their independent living apartments and provide services as needed.

Retirement communities can usually provide contact information for agencies that some of their residents use.

These services are divided into two buckets: medical and non-medical. Generally, nurses provide medical services. Aides provide other kinds of services.

For example, some of the services listed by one agency are: walking the dog, preparing meals, running errands, going grocery shopping, helping manage the calendar so that people don't miss appointments, helping with mail, and going with individuals to their doctors' appointments.

Residents pay for such services a la carte, instead of having much of their care simply bundled into the monthly fees that they pay to the retirement community. It is more work for the resident or representative to manage.

It can be less expensive if relatively little help is needed. It can be more expensive if a great deal of care is required. But it is certainly an option, especially in the short term.

Some people simply don't want to move—they like their independent living apartments and want to stay there. Nothing (except possibly money and the need to manage the situation) stops them from bringing in services from the outside day after day, year after year.

Care management in this case is no different from what it would be if you were living in your own house. Nothing stops you from arranging any kind of care you want or need to bring in, assuming that you can pay for it.

Moving from one level of assisted living care to another level that the retirement community is licensed to provide does not require any additional moves. That is, you do not need to change apartments as you need more of the assisted living services that the site offers.

Alta Vista's license covers two levels of assisted living care but not the third and highest level of assisted living licensing that the state offers, called "directed care." Good Samaritan, Granite Gate, and Las Fuentes are all licensed to provide all three levels of care.

Next week's column will talk about what happens if you need a level of care that exceeds the unit's license. That is, it will cover what happens at Alta Vista if you come to need care beyond the second level of assisted living, and what happens in all four organizations if it turns out that you need long term nursing/skilled nursing care (also sometimes termed "nursing home" or "long-term care" services).

10

Moving From Assisted Living To Nursing/Skilled Nursing

What if you're in assisted living in a retirement community and you need more care?

One option is to move to a building in your retirement community where the type of care you need is offered. For example, Good Samaritan and Las Fuentes both offer nursing/skilled nursing facilities in addition to assisted living units.

If your community doesn't offer that level of care—Granite Gate and Alta Vista don't offer nursing/skilled nursing facilities, for example—then a second option is to move to a different retirement community's unit that offers that level of care, or to leave retirement communities entirely and move to a freestanding long-term care facility (nursing home).

Moving to Las Fuentes or Good Samaritan in Prescott from Alta Vista isn't geographically a big move. All three communities are within shouting distance of each other.

Although it would require a little bit of effort on the part of your family or friends left behind, it should not be too difficult for them to come see you. Granite Gate is further away.

But suppose that you very much like your assisted living apartment and don't want to move.

Or suppose that you are half of a couple, and only one of you needs skilled nursing.

You might find it very expensive to pay for two separate homes, one an apartment in assisted living and one a room in a skilled nursing unit. Even if you have the money to pay for two homes, perhaps the two of you don't want to live apart.

Then you might consider a third option, which is to stay in assisted living and bring supplemental skilled nursing services in from outside the retirement community to your apartment.

The law prohibits a facility that is licensed to provide assisted living from providing skilled nursing services to you that it isn't licensed to provide.

However, the law does not prohibit you (or your representatives) from independently making arrangements with an organization such as a nursing agency to come in and provide additional services to you.

The law does put half a dozen hoops in your way, but they do not seem very hard to jump through. For example, you may have to get a note signed by your doctor saying that she agrees that you can safely stay in the assisted living unit.

You or your representative may have to sign a document saying that you understand the limits of the assisted living services provided and explicitly saying that you want to stay in assisted living anyway. And so forth.

It is less clear that this strategy is workable at Alta Vista, which is licensed to provide the first and second levels of assisted living care, but not the third level.

Assisted living units licensed to provide "personal care" (the second level) are forbidden by law from having people living in them who require "directed care" (the third level). Nursing home care is typically a level beyond the third level of assisted living care.

Alta Vista points out that residents could revert to independent living status, and arrange to get all services from outside agencies, in order to stay there.

That approach is possible, although it sounds to me as if it might be cumbersome. If you are interested in Alta Vista, talk to its management about this topic, because individual circumstances and solutions can vary, and the law is complex.

If you've moved into a skilled nursing facility, does that mean that you're done moving? Not necessarily.

If you develop dementia and become hostile or threatening to other residents, or you start to wander away and don't know how to find your way back or even how to ask for help, you might have to move again, to a memory care unit specifically set up to handle such situations.

What's the key point? Before you decide to move to a retirement community, it's important to understand clearly what care you can—and cannot—expect to get there, and what other arrangements you might eventually need to make to get some types of care.

II

Examples

This section describes retirement communities operated by four organizations in the Prescott, AZ area.

One of these, Good Samaritan, operates two campuses with some similar and some different services at each. For simplicity's sake, I sometimes refer to four communities, combining the two Good Samaritan locations.

11

Las Fuentes Resort Village

Las Fuentes offers independent living, assisted living, and nursing/skilled nursing care.

Las Fuentes is a fun place to be.

Outings to jazz concerts, casinos, golf chipping, and dozens of other events and activities are offered. Liz Schmidt, Sales Director, commented, "If a new restaurant opens in Prescott, within two months we've taken a busload of residents there."

Saturday nights typically find residents enjoying the "stationary cruise ship," with live entertainment and entrees such as prime rib.

Residents volunteer to run activities; one example is a "Write Your Life" course that helped interested residents create autobiographies. Crafts, cooking, Bible study, and dozens of other activities are available.

Garden beds raised to hip height allow people in wheelchairs the chance to get involved in an activity that most people assume must be done kneeling on the ground.

Las Fuentes offers residents many chances to volunteer. Near Christmas, a number of residents buy gifts that needy seniors outside of Las Fuentes wish for.

A food collection box seems to be a permanent fixture in the lobby. The Knit & Chat group knits booties and blankets for babies born in the hospital nearby.

With 290 residents, Las Fuentes is able to attract politicians such as Governor Jan Brewer to come speak, especially in the run-up to elections.

Las Fuentes feels spacious, from the soaring lobby and a three-story atrium to its 16 acres—including a one-acre cottonwood park with paths and benches—and apartments with walk-in pantries and sizes that range up to about 1700 square feet.

Most of its independent living apartments have their own patios or balconies. It is the only site I toured that offers underground parking.

It has three full-time drivers, who travel regular routes to take people to grocery stores, the post office, banks, the public library, and doctors' appointments.

Resident Services—separate from the Activities department—has an office on the lower level. This group provides orientation for all new residents. Its staff visits residents in the hospital, and will take care of mail, plants, etc. until they come home.

Resident Services provides information for the in-house cable channel that announces birthdays and anniversaries (if residents agree), as well as specials in the dining room.

A copy machine is free to residents. Several free washers and dryers are found in laundry rooms on each floor, often allowing people to get multiple loads done at the same time.

The bustling lobby is staffed by a receptionist 24/7. Schmidt explained, "If somebody comes in and doesn't know your apartment number, we won't let them past the desk unless we reach you in your apartment and you say that it's okay to let them up. We take resident security very seriously."

A number of staff members have been there since Las Fuentes opened its doors 16 years ago. "We know what works with our residents. We provide continuity of care over the years," Schmidt noted.

Its parent company, Century Park Associates, manages 42 independent and assisted living communities across the country, according to its website. Its affiliate, Life Care Centers of America, manages hundreds of nursing homes.

Schmidt commented, "This management company won't back out or change. They've never sold a single one of their facilities."

Catching up with a table of residents at the wildly popular Thursday buffet, I found the group so lively that it was hard to keep up with their comments.

Asked what they liked best about living at Las Fuentes, the answers came tumbling out, and were variations on a few themes: they love all the friends they've made; they find the people—both residents and staff—friendly and helpful; and they enjoy the wide variety of activities available to them.

Asked what they would change at Las Fuentes if they could wave a magic wand, the energetic and enthusiastic group falls silent. They take the question seriously and think hard. Then the consensus is, "Nothing stands out," and "Everything runs smoothly."

12

Alta Vista

Elegance. Enter the lobby of Alta Vista, and the first thing you see is a massive, intricate hardwood spiral staircase rising to the heavens. The outfitting of the rest of the site is consistent with that first image. Fireplaces are grand. Artwork is stunning. Hallways are impressive.

Even the bathrooms have granite counters, as does the massive kitchen in the activities room, which in most retirement communities is almost certain to be made of Formica.

Alta Vista is easily the most upscale of the four retirement communities visited for this series. The impression created is more "4-star resort hotel" than "retirement community."

The dining options follow suit. It is typical in some retirement communities for the restaurant to offer two main entrees. At Alta Vista, the menu looks closer to that of an upscale restaurant.

A recent dinner menu offered "Light Fare" including two soups, chili, two salads, a quesadilla, crab cakes, boneless chicken wings, and charred pork tenderloin.

The "Specialties" on that menu included filet mignon, fresh Atlantic salmon, grilled chicken breast, shrimp scampi, and a classic burger.

While there is a restaurant in the assisted living wing, its residents are welcome to eat in the main restaurant as well.

Independent living apartments offer both a regular stove/oven and a built-in microwave above the stove. Both independent and assisted living apartments offer granite counters and cherry hardwood cabinets in the kitchen.

Every apartment includes a stacked clothes washer/dryer. One staff member commented, "We've signed so many contracts because of the washer/dryers! That's a feature that potential residents really care about."

A large patio provides quite a few tables, chairs, and benches to permit leisurely enjoyment of the fine view of Thumb Butte and other scenery.

When asked what distinguishes Alta Vista, Executive Director Maggie Greenwood immediately replied, "We truly offer a lifestyle of choices. We have a motto: We don't say no, we say, 'How can we make this work?'"

Recent activities offered, in addition to those typical of most retirement communities, included swimming at

Yavapai College, scenic drives, karaoke, cooking demos, a harp concert, a winetasting at a local vineyard, a Corvette car show, and a wealth management seminar.

When asked what they liked most, residents replied, "Wonderful facility," "Food is excellent," "People are friendly," "Staff is good to us," and "We feel safe."

One resident spoke in glowing terms of one of the chefs who regularly comes out of the kitchen and talks with residents in both restaurants.

"He obviously enjoys his work, chatting with his guests, learns how his food is received and welcomes suggestions. He is so dedicated to pleasing his diners that he will make time to make something special for you, like the mushroom gravy he prepares for me for my steak and the extra mushrooms for my wife, as he has found out she thoroughly enjoys mushrooms with any entrée."

The resident concluded, "Dining in either of the two dining rooms at Alta Vista is a pleasure," and this chef is "a treasure."

When asked what they'd like to see change, residents' first answer, slow in coming, was, "That's a tough question."

Alta Vista's newness can be an advantage—the physical plant is exquisite and will likely remain that way for some time. It also raises a note of caution: this retirement community has been open for only about a year and a half.

As with many businesses, it's simply not possible to predict how it would fare if there were another economic downturn or other challenges.

Its current management company has a long history in the assisted living business. Based on its history, it also appears to have a tendency to move on to other projects after a few years. You may decide that Alta Vista has so many appealing features that it's worth considering regardless.

13

Granite Gate Senior Living

Granite Gate is set in the magnificent rocks of Granite Dells. There are no bad views from the windows of Granite Gate. Common rooms and dining rooms with soaring ceilings and floor-to-ceiling glass windows make the most of the scenery.

When people move in to Granite Gate—even into independent living—they start getting some services right away that are more typical of assisted living.

For example, all meals are automatically included. Further, people don't need to change apartments if they start out in independent living and later need assisted living services.

Perhaps because of these features, its residents tend to be 5-10 years older than those in the other retirement communities I visited for this series.

If residents later develop advanced dementia, they can move into Granite Gate's dedicated memory care unit (space permitting).

Granite Gate does not offer skilled nursing, so residents who need this type of care might move elsewhere.

However, Executive Director Rena Phillips pointed out that families often bring in specialized outside services, such as wound care or hospice care, so that their aging relatives can stay in the apartments that have become their homes.

Granite Gate offers apartments of up to 1400 square feet, which means that people getting assisted living services have homes that are unusually spacious for this level of care.

Residents are often very active and involved. One resident stands behind the bar at happy hour, offering punch and little cups of mixed nuts to fellow residents.

Other residents can be seen on stage in talent shows and other performances, while fellow residents form an appreciative audience.

Granite Gate offers many activities typical of retirement communities, as well as several not mentioned elsewhere, such as a Cookies & Conversation Club and a Walking Club.

What do the residents have to say?

A number of them told me that their families found Granite Gate for them, and that they love it there.

One reported, "It is very pleasant here. Everyone is cooperative and friendly. It's in a beautiful setting. We checked out quite a few places. It's excellent. They take care of everything beautifully. They don't let things go; they take care of everything right away."

Another resident commented, "I love the independence I have here. I come and go as I please. It's homey. They make you feel very much at home. The staff is wonderful. They all take beautiful care of me. It's a beautiful building. We have very good transportation. It's a nice clientele of people here. You can be active or be in your room."

Another resident's face lit up as if she had been handed the best present in the world when I asked her what she liked most about living there.

She said, "Everyone here is so kind and gentle. Residents and employees are wonderful people. After my husband died, I just didn't know how I'd get along, but I'm very, very comfortable. You know, when you watch TV, it always has bad news—but it doesn't penetrate here. It's just a wonderful, wonderful place. We looked at four places before choosing this one. I just fell in love with the apartment. I don't know a single person who could say anything negative about it."

When asked what they would want to change, one resident suggested more benches outside, an improvement that Phillips reported was already under way.

The community has had three different owners in about the last six years. Current owners, Five Star Quality Care, took over in May 2011 and immediately made a number of improvements. Sometimes, though, their corporate communication can raise questions for visitors. For example, prominently posted are the Five Star Values, the *fourth* of which is "Put People First." If the intention is to put people first, why isn't that the first value?

But when I checked the results of state licensing inspections, Granite Gate had the best inspection results of the four organizations I looked into. If resident comments and state inspection records are anything to go by, Granite Gate certainly does put people first.

14

Good Samaritan

Good Samaritan has heart.

Owned by the Evangelical Lutheran Good Samaritan Society, it is the only nonprofit among the four retirement communities I looked into in the area. Good Samaritan reports that it is the largest nonprofit provider of senior care communities in the country.

Its vision is "to create an environment where people are loved, valued and at peace."

It makes a compelling case that it does just that. Staff members with whom I spoke uniformly appeared passionate and committed. They were excited to talk about changes underway to improve the environment for their residents.

Cindy Brown, Relationship Development Director, reported that employees are explicitly told, "You will never be disciplined or taken aside and talked to because you took the time to listen to a resident, to talk with a resident."

The community is divided into segments that tend to be relatively small. For example, in Prescott Valley (its newer campus, about 15 years old) it has space for 28 people in independent living, 16 people in memory care, 20 people in its short-term rehabilitation unit, and 44 people in long-term skilled nursing.

Smaller units mean that staff and residents get to know each other and build relationships that would be harder to develop in larger units. Residents seem to have a sense that they are home. Its sites offer multiple little nooks and crannies, little parlors and sitting areas that are nicely appointed and welcoming.

Good Samaritan offers a range of activities similar to those at other retirement communities. It also lists some unique offerings. A recent calendar for Willow Wind, its assisted living unit, listed balloon volleyball, a group crossword puzzle, games such as Yahtzee and Skip-Bo, and a Lucille Ball marathon.

Wii fitness games are popular here, as they are in most retirement communities.

In a couple parts of Good Samaritan, I saw residents interact with dogs trained to provide pet therapy. Residents' faces lit up as they petted and talked with the animals.

Good Samaritan has a choir and other musical groups. It offers the services of a chaplain and makes a serious effort to meet the various spiritual needs of its residents, stressing that it welcomes people of any (or no) religious beliefs. It offers religious services of various denominations.

The walls sport paintings provided by the Mountain Artists Guild in Prescott and by the Prescott Valley Art Guild in Prescott Valley, local artists' groups. The displays are changed regularly and the artwork is available for purchase.

Every year Good Samaritan hires an independent company to survey its residents, to get feedback about how the residents feel about living there.

Its assisted living unit is striking for the great thought that has gone into its design. I was particularly charmed to see a vast vegetable garden in a safe interior courtyard.

Residents are helped to grow large bumper crops of dozens of vegetables. These are then incorporated into their meals, which are prepared almost entirely from scratch by their chef.

What do residents like best? The small size of the units they belong to, decent food, and the fellowship they experience with other residents—a sense of family. The immediate answer, when asked what they would change? "Not a thing."

Good Samaritan offers the most comprehensive array of services of the four organizations visited for this series.

On its Prescott campus, it offers independent living in casitas and in apartments, assisted living, long-term care (nursing/skilled nursing), short-term rehab, inpatient hospice care and inpatient hospice respite care—as well as HUD-subsidized senior housing. It also offers home health care and home-based hospice care.

In Prescott Valley, it offers independent living apartments, long-term care (nursing/skilled nursing), short-term rehab, and an Alzheimer's/dementia care unit.

Good Samaritan does not have one central phone number to call locally and it can be difficult to find contact information for some parts of the organization.

Readers interested in Good Samaritan are welcome to call Cindy Brown in Good Samaritan's administrative offices at (928) 443-9760 ext. 39707. She has volunteered to help readers navigate the extensive—but bewildering—array of options that Good Samaritan offers.

III

Costs

Figuring out how to pay the costs for living in a retirement community can seem daunting. This section provides examples of costs in the area—and explains how you might cover the bill.

15

Costs: Independent Living
and Assisted Living

In other parts of the country, people sometimes have to pay hundreds of thousands of dollars to buy into a retirement community.

The good news in Prescott is that none of the four retirement communities I looked into requires a big upfront fee. The financial arrangements are simpler—closer to renting an apartment than to buying a house.

Annual costs for one person in a mid-sized independent living apartment, including meals, follow. (Apartment name and square footage are in parentheses.)

Good Samaritan (Windsong Villas in Prescott Valley, 849 sf): $27,000; Las Fuentes (Bedford, 915 sf): $40,000; Granite Gate (Cottonwood, 846 sf): $43,000; Alta Vista (Premier Suite, 841 sf): $48,000.

A few notes: Good Samaritan includes 20 lunches a month in its rates and encourages residents to take home extra soup and salad for dinner; I added $250/month for groceries to cover other meals.

At Granite Gate, all meals are included. At Alta Vista, I've added the cost of a full meal plan, at $400/month. At Las Fuentes, I've added $490/month to cover all full meals.

At Alta Vista and Las Fuentes, one may also buy individual meals. At Las Fuentes, another option is to buy smaller (and less expensive) breakfasts and/or lunches.

The costs for a second person in the apartment are typically either simply the cost of meals, or the cost of meals plus $150-$250/month. Annually, these numbers work out to roughly $5000 to $8000 for a second person.

If you look at the numbers and gulp, two points may help. First, remember that I have included food costs. Second, understand that the totals may not be as different from your expenses today as they first appear. Worksheets offered by Alta Vista and Las Fuentes show why.

They provide space for you to write in your costs today for items such as rent/mortgage, homeowners' insurance, property taxes, homeowners' association fees, housecleaning, cable TV, electricity, water/sewer, gas/heating, lawn care, snow removal, pest control, garbage removal, home maintenance, and transportation.

Then in the column for your expenses in the retirement community, after each of these items (except rent), it says, "Included."

You may see it differently for some of the items. For example, you may want to keep your car. Perhaps you want more cable stations than their package includes. While you may not need homeowners' insurance, you may want renters' insurance.

On the other hand, your costs could be lower than the examples suggest, because you may decide that you need less space and can therefore choose a smaller, less expensive apartment.

For example, knowing that you can entertain guests in the restaurant onsite—or even in a private dining room—you may conclude that having a large dining area in your apartment is unnecessary.

The lowest cost apartments are as much as $15,000 less expensive than the above examples; including meals (and in Good Samaritan's case, an adjustment adding $450 for groceries since no meals are included at this site) these lowest cost apartments are: Good Samaritan (one bedroom in Prescott, 480 sf): $22,000; Granite Gate (Willow, 480 sf): $28,000; Las Fuentes (Chester, 605 sf): $32,000; Alta Vista (Ambassador Suite, 605 sf): $35,000.

Assisted living apartments are typically smaller than independent living apartments (except at Granite Gate, where every apartment/bed in the community is licensed for assisted living). State law requires that even the lowest level of assisted living include three meals a day plus a snack.

The base rates for typical assisted living units are about as follows: Granite Gate (Chaparral, 564 sf):

$30,000; Alta Vista (Gold Suite, 571 sf): $39,000; Good Samaritan (two bedroom, 608+ sf): $40,000; Las Fuentes (one bedroom, 576 sf): $45,000. Smaller apartments are offered in each community at a lower cost.

Each community is careful to point out that additional assisted living charges are likely to apply, depending on the individual's specific needs.

These charges may be relatively modest (say, $150/month) or extensive (say, $1800/month). You can ask the communities you are interested in to estimate the costs for any specific case you have in mind.

The least expensive sites for independent living are not necessarily the same as those for assisted living.

16

Costs: Nursing/Skilled Nursing and Memory Care

The facilities included here are part of retirement communities in the Prescott area run by Good Samaritan, Granite Gate, and Las Fuentes.

According to the United States Department of Health and Human Services (HHS), 70 percent of people age 65-plus will need long-term care at some point in their lives.

More than 40 percent will need the care offered in a nursing home, where average costs in the U.S. are about $84,000/year for a private room. A semi-private room (housing two people) costs about $75,000/year per person.

Depending on the level of care needed, a bed in a semi-private room at Good Samaritan costs $73,000-86,000/year, and private rooms cost $81,000-95,000/year.

The private rooms in Good Samaritan are the same size as the rooms that house two people.

The rates for a bed in a two-person room at Las Fuentes start at $75,000/year, very small private rooms start at $85,000/year, and private rooms the size of the rooms that house two people start at $135,000/year.

In all cases, the rates at Las Fuentes may be significantly higher than those noted here depending on the level of care needed.

Comparing apples to apples, Good Samaritan costs less than Las Fuentes for basic long-term care. For an individual in a large private room, in fact, the costs are about $54,000 less at Good Samaritan than at Las Fuentes.

You can ask each organization to tell you its price for any specific situation you have in mind, since charges for added services can vary significantly.

Costs for memory care at Good Samaritan are $83,000/year for a semi-private room and $92,000/year for a private room.

At Granite Gate, costs for memory care are about $58,000/year for a semi-private apartment and $84,000/year for a private apartment. The Granite Gate apartments are quite a bit larger than the rooms at Good Samaritan.

Charges for memory care in both communities cover all levels of care offered. That is, unlike the case in other long-term care units (assisted living and nursing/skilled nursing), rates are not tiered based on the intensity of services provided by the facility.

Good Samaritan's memory care unit is licensed as a nursing/skilled nursing facility, while Granite Gate's is licensed for assisted living. Thus, the services offered may not be identical. It is reasonable to find out if all the services you need are included, and to ask for a cost estimate if additional outside services might be needed.

Note that I have converted all the costs in this article into annual numbers. However, long-term care facilities typically charge by the day or by the month. That is, when an individual stops using the services, charges stop either that day or in the worst case, at the end of the month.

None of the numbers quoted above include what might be called standard medical expenses—doctors' visits, prescription drugs, lab tests, eyeglasses, some types of medical supplies, and so forth. In addition, the numbers quoted don't include personal expenses, such as clothing or toiletries.

The rates at Good Samaritan do include expenses for ancillary equipment that some people need, such as wheelchairs or walkers.

Many people assume that Medicare will cover the costs of nursing homes. However, with the exception of a short period after a hospitalization, generally Medicare will not cover these costs.

The sheer size of these numbers can be startling if this is the first time you have looked at them. You might be wondering how you could possibly pay these rates.

One point to keep in mind is that people do not typically need this level of service for decades. In fact, according to HHS, typically "someone who is 65 today will need some type of long-term care services and supports for three years." And 80 percent need services for less than five years.

The next column will talk about some ways to find the money to cover the costs of living in a retirement community. As is true for covering the costs of college, quite a few different options are available, and you might be surprised to discover some that you hadn't considered.

17

Covering Costs:
Independent Living

Costs for an independent living apartment and meals for one person in communities researched for this series range from $22,000/year to $62,000/year, depending on the community and on the apartment size.

For two people, the cost is generally increased by roughly the cost of meals for a second person. Occasionally, there is a relatively small additional monthly fee unrelated to meals.

So how can you cover the costs?

Retirement communities are typically happy to help you find answers to this question. They may have an expert onsite, or they may refer you to a third party who can help you work through the numbers at no charge.

Solutions for a 65-year-old in good health may be different from those for an 85-year-old in poor health. That said, four common options for paying for independent living follow.

First, use money you currently spend on living expenses that will go away with a move to a retirement community.

These include items such as rent/mortgage, homeowners' insurance, utilities, house cleaning, building and grounds maintenance, perhaps automobile expenses and insurance, and meals if you have included the cost of meals in the retirement community calculation.

Additionally, remember to include big periodic expenses, such as roof repairs, plumbing and electrical repairs, major kitchen appliance replacements, and so forth.

If you include the cost of a meal plan in your numbers, you might also find that you can apply money that you have typically spent on restaurants to your total costs in the retirement community; you may "eat out" in the onsite restaurant every day and feel less need to leave the campus to go to other restaurants.

You may also find that you spend less on entertainment, since you can enjoy many activities and entertainments offered at no extra charge.

Second, if you sell a house as part of a move, you might spend some of the resulting money (or the income it generates when invested) each year.

For example, if you sold your house for $200,000 and you and your financial planner (if you have one) agree that it is reasonable to spend 4 percent of that money each year, you could apply $8000/year to the costs of the retirement community.

A financial planner will generally expect that growth in your diversified portfolio will more than cover this withdrawal, typically leaving you with at least as much money at the end of the year as you had at the beginning.

Third, consider using some of your assets to buy an immediate fixed annuity. In exchange for purchasing the annuity, you are promised monthly payments for life, starting right away. Some people consider buying an annuity to be akin to creating a pension for themselves.

In this scenario, depending on your age and the interest rates in effect, you may end up with more money to spend each month than you would by simply drawing 4 percent of the value of your investments each year.

Fourth, consider buying "longevity insurance," which is how some people describe a deferred fixed annuity. For example, you might buy an annuity at age 60 that would start making monthly payments to you when you are 75, to coincide with a planned move into a retirement community.

This approach, like that involving immediate annuities, could provide more cash than you would otherwise feel safe spending, given your assets.

It is critical to consult a competent financial advisor before considering any of these options except the first, because each comes with serious pitfalls that can cause you big problems if you are not extremely familiar with them.

For example, if you turn over a chunk of your assets to an insurance company that goes bankrupt, you could lose virtually all of the money that you put into an annuity.

As another example, if it is important to you to have the greatest amount of money possible to give to your heirs, then you might not want to use some of it to buy an annuity.

Further, if you buy an annuity when interest rates are low, it may not provide as much income as you thought it would, and it is possible that you would have ended up with more money to spend by keeping it yourself in a diversified portfolio.

Each solution also has tax implications that should be understood before you proceed.

The next column will talk about ways to pay for assisted living and skilled nursing.

18

Covering Costs:
Assisted Living and Long-Term Care

Costs for basic assisted living for one person at sites studied for this series range from $28,000 to $56,000/year. A second person will add from $6000 to $16,000/year.

Additional services can add $2000 to $20,000 per person per year. And long-term care (nursing home) and skilled nursing care can cost from $73,000 to well over $100,000 per person per year.

What options are available to cover the costs?

The four options mentioned in the previous article about independent living costs apply here: using the money that would have gone into a mortgage and other home expenses, drawing a small percentage every year of the money from the sale of a home, buying an immediate fixed annuity, and buying a deferred fixed annuity.

Five additional options follow.

Long-term care insurance. Consider purchasing long-term care insurance when you are still relatively young and healthy—perhaps in your mid-50s.

Kenneth Stephenson, a Chartered Financial Consultant who runs Complete Financial Solutions in North Carolina, pointed out that such insurance can help protect the rest of your assets.

Tax deductions. Look into deducting assisted living and long-term care expenses on federal and state tax returns.

Costs for assisted living can typically be considered medical expenses for tax purposes if there is a clear medical reason for the level of care received.

Costs for nursing care can almost always be counted as medical expenses.

Under one scenario for tax laws going forward, medical expenses that exceed 10 percent of your adjusted gross income could generally be deducted, assuming that you collect the paperwork needed to support the deduction. Someone with $50,000 in income could generally deduct medical expenses beyond the first $5000.

The practical effect of the tax deduction is that, for example, a couple with $100,000 in adjusted gross income and $70,000 in assisted living expenses might eliminate federal and state tax on $60,000 (the deduction for medical expenses that exceed 10 percent of adjusted gross income).

That deduction might free up roughly $8000 to $27,000 that would otherwise have gone to taxes, depending on many factors such as the sources of the couple's income and their other deductions.

Accelerated life insurance benefits. Look into taking accelerated life insurance benefits, available with some types of life insurance policies if life expectancy is relatively short. In this situation, the insurer pays some or all of the insurance benefits to you while you are still alive.

Veterans Aid & Attendance Pension Benefit. Find out if you are eligible for the U.S. Department of Veterans Affairs' Aid & Attendance Pension Benefit, available to veterans with limited assets who served during wartime and/or their spouses.

The income ceiling is about $20,000/year, but as noted at www.payingforseniorcare.com, "The VA allows individuals to deduct their out-of-pocket medical expenses [such as] health insurance premiums, assisted living, home care and adult day care costs from their income."

For example, if you pay $50,000 for assisted living and your income is $60,000, you might still qualify. Maximum benefits range from about $13,000 to $24,000/year.

Medicaid. Check into state Medicaid funding, available if assets and income fall below certain limits. In Arizona, the program is named Arizona Long Term Care System (ALTCS).

An individual's income must be under about $25,000 to be eligible; a couple's income limit is twice that. This resource may pay most of the cost of essential care in some cases.

Retirement communities typically can direct you to people who can help you figure out—at no charge—what funding sources might help in your case and how to apply.

Another resource is www.payingforseniorcare.com.

Its Resource Locator Tool offers an online questionnaire and then provides a very comprehensive report listing what sources of funds may be available, given the individual's or couple's particular financial and medical circumstances.

Every type of funding listed above comes with quite a few cautionary notes and fine print details that you might be tempted to skip—but doing so could result in unpleasant surprises.

That's why it is important to get competent advice before committing to decisions that would be hard to reverse.

The next column will talk about the financial profile of people who move into retirement communities. How much do they have in assets? What is their typical income?

It will also explain the financial arrangements at retirement communities in Phoenix and in other parts of the country that require large upfront fees, in case you are considering such a community for yourself or for aging relatives who live elsewhere.

19

Do You Have To Be Wealthy To Live In a Retirement Community?

Costs to live in the communities studied for this series can range from $22,000/year to well over $100,000/year, depending on the community, the size of the room or apartment, and any medical attention needed.

None of these communities requires a big upfront fee, but about two-thirds of the retirement communities around the country that offer a full range of services do.

Because you may consider such a community in Phoenix or elsewhere, or have aging relatives in other parts of the country where such fees are common, I'll explain this model.

Such full-service communities are termed Continuing Care Retirement Communities (CCRCs). AARP reports, "CCRCs guarantee lifetime housing, social activities and increased levels of care as needs change" and they "require a hefty entrance fee . . .[ranging] from $100,000 to $1 million."

According to industry sources, the average is about $248,000. Do you have to be wealthy to consider any retirement community, much less one that charges big entrance fees?

As of 2009, according to an industry report provided by Angela Green, Regional Sales Manager for Seniority, Inc., a national senior living consulting group, about half the residents in CCRCs had annual household incomes of less than $50,000.

Nearly half of new residents had a net worth of under $300,000. (Net worth is the value of assets such as investments and/or a house less any debts or loans, such as a mortgage and/or credit card debt.)

Tom Dorough, Executive Director of a CCRC called The Terraces of Phoenix, explained that most residents use the money from the sale of a home to pay the entrance fee, and then use pensions, social security, retirement accounts and other investments and the income they generate to pay the monthly fees.

CCRCs such as The Terraces of Phoenix work hard to help address people's fears that they will run out of money. As is typical with such communities, potential residents undergo a comprehensive financial and medical review.

A computer model uses information about their health, age, assets, and income to estimate how long they are likely to live, how long their money will last, and how much money they will have left in their estates.

Many CCRCs accept only residents who are able to live independently when they apply to enter. And not surprisingly, only people who are likely to be able to pay their bills are offered entrance.

Green, from the consulting company, commented, "Studies show that people who live in retirement communities actually spend less time in assisted living or long-term care, because they stay healthier and more active. That has tremendous financial benefits, because independent living is less expensive."

But occasionally, individuals are caught short by unexpectedly large expenses due to extended stays in long-term care or skilled nursing units. What happens then? Green explained, "Most nonprofit CCRCs commit to keeping people even if they run out of money. It is part of our mission."

Dorough, the CCRC executive, noted, "This commitment applies if residents' financial resources are depleted through no fault of their own. People may outlive their assets, and living in a CCRC ensures that even if this happens, their health care and lifestyle are still guaranteed."

Green pointed out that moving into a CCRC that operates under this model could be considered akin to buying a form of long-term care insurance.

That is, everyone in the community contributes by paying a large upfront fee, and then a few people whose care ends up being considerably more expensive than anticipated are covered by funds the community has collected, even if those few individuals can't pay their bills.

The extensive medical and financial evaluation is a point of difference between the typical CCRC and the communities reviewed here in Prescott.

While a medical review may be done at communities here for the purposes of placing people in the right level of care, people may enter at any level that meets their needs and has space available.

Financial reviews are far less extensive, and may be limited to credit checks and other standard reviews that consumers may experience before signing any consumer contract.

IV

Other Housing Options

If retirement communities don't meet your needs, another option is a freestanding assisted living or skilled nursing/nursing facility (nursing home) when help is needed with daily care.

If retirement communities sound appealing but are outside your price range, one alternative is housing whose rent is subsidized by the federal government.

In Prescott, another alternative is a unique state-subsidized retirement home for long-time residents.

20

Freestanding Assisted Living and Long-Term Care Facilities

Previous articles profiled retirement communities in the Prescott area that each offer a range of living options.

For people unable to live independently, another choice is a standalone facility that offers assisted living or skilled nursing/nursing care. Nursing facilities may also be called nursing homes or long-term care facilities.

Costs appear similar to those for similar levels of care in retirement communities.

Arizona allows for assisted living *centers* (licensed for more than 10 residents and usually housing 50-100 people) and assisted living *homes* (licensed for 10 or fewer residents).

Standalone assisted living centers that offer dementia care include the Margaret T. Morris Center and Highgate Senior Living. (Highgate also offers regular assisted living.)

A few additional freestanding assisted living centers operate in the area. In addition, there are more than 20 local assisted living homes, housing 5-10 residents each.

Several freestanding nursing/skilled nursing facilities locally have space for about 65-115 residents each.

It is beyond the scope of this column to evaluate all standalone facilities. However, I can tell you the steps I would take if I were researching facilities for a relative:

1. Identify available options.
2. Look at their state inspection results.
3. Check out their websites.
4. Visit the facilities in person.
5. Compare the sites.

Identify available options. One source for a list of facilities is the licensing website of the Arizona Department of Health and Human Services, which can be found at http://www.azdhs.gov/als/databases/index.htm.

The listings are organized into categories such as assisted living, long-term care, etc. and sorted by zip code.

The assisted living list separates out sites by license level: directed care, personal care, and supervisory care. Directed care is the highest level of licensing available for assisted living facilities in Arizona.

Look at their state inspection results. At http://www.azdhs.gov/als/, select Facility Search and then the type of care (for example, assisted living) and search on the facility's name.

Virtually every assisted living and skilled nursing/long-term care facility gets citations (notices of problems) as a result of inspections.

The regulations are lengthy and complex, and perfection is hard to come by. The question to ask is whether the citations suggest that residents are at risk.

For example, health care workers generally must be tested to prove that they are free of tuberculosis when they start work and once a year after that, according to state law.

Suppose that a new employee had the test six months earlier at another employer, and then got the test on day 2 instead of on day 1 with the current employer, and both tests showed that she did not have tuberculosis.

Because she did not have the test day 1, the facility is in violation of the law and may get a citation. But it seems unlikely that residents were at risk.

Now consider an example that might lead you to a different conclusion.

The state generally requires that employees involved in direct patient care get a fingerprint clearance card, which indicates that the state has concluded that they have not been convicted of homicide, sexual assault, and so forth.

If a facility gets a citation for continuing to employ a worker who has been denied a fingerprint clearance card, you might be concerned on two counts:

For one, might vulnerable residents be at risk? For another, if management violates this regulation, are they similarly lax about other important requirements? Don't assume that inspectors will have discovered every problem.

Check out their websites. Once you have created a short list of facilities whose type, location and inspection records look acceptable to you, read their websites. If facilities don't have websites, it raises questions for me about their communication strategies.

Visit the facilities in person. Take checklists so that you remember to ask questions important to you. One site that offers very detailed checklists about costs and contracts, personal care, quality of life, and so forth is www.caregiverslibrary.org under Checklists & Forms. Trust your senses and intuition during your visit.

Compare the sites. Your list may be shorter now, and it is time to compare the sites you are still considering—on characteristics that are important to the prospective resident. I was reminded of this point when I described local retirement communities to an older relative in terms of apartment size, meal options, amenities and activities. She replied, "I don't care about any of that. As long as I can get cheese and coffee, all I care about is having great internet access."

The next two columns will discuss subsidized senior housing, which may be an excellent choice if money is quite limited.

21

Subsidized Housing: What Is It?

Readers living on limited incomes may find that retirement communities discussed in previous articles are out of reach.

An alternative is very affordable apartments available to people age 62-plus through programs run by the U.S. Department of Housing and Urban Development (HUD).

Residents in HUD-subsidized apartments pay a relatively small portion of the rent that their apartments would command on the open market; the federal government pays the rest.

Three sites visited for this article are Casa de Pinos (run by Retirement Housing Foundation, affiliated with the United Church of Christ), Village Tower (run by the Evangelical Lutheran Good Samaritan Society), and Bradshaw Senior Community.

The first two run under one type of HUD program often referred to as Section 8 housing; Bradshaw operates under a different federal program, called Section 42, which has somewhat different rules and requirements. I'll describe the financial arrangements for the first two first.

Each apartment complex has a different contract with HUD that specifies how many apartments can be rented to people with "low income," "very low income," and "extremely low income."

At both Casa de Pinos and Village Tower, only people with "very low income" (for 2013 in Yavapai County, under $19,250/year) and "extremely low income" (under $11,550/year) qualify for apartments at this time.

The income limits are established separately for every county, so people who qualify in one county might not qualify in another.

The limits are adjusted upwards—although not by much—for larger households. For two people, the household income limit for the "very low income" category is $22,000 and for the "extremely low income" category, the limit is $13,200.

Assets are considered, but people do not have to use up all of their assets ("spend down") to qualify.

Depending on several variables, HUD calculations consider either the actual income from assets (interest, dividends, etc.) or assume that they provide income equal to 2 percent of the assets' market value.

That is, if someone owns stock worth $100,000, then under the 2 percent approach, $2000 would be added to their annual income from other sources such as Social Security, pensions, and so forth, to come up with their total income.

Suppose that Linda has $15,000 in total income. Assuming that she is a U.S. citizen or eligible immigrant, that she passes a background check, and that an apartment is available, she would be eligible to rent a subsidized apartment.

At Casa de Pinos and Village Tower, the rent charged is limited to 30 percent of the residents' adjusted income.

The calculation is more complex than you might assume, because potential residents are permitted to subtract out some allowances and expenses to get to the adjusted income used to determine their rent.

For example, medical expenses in excess of 3 percent of income can be subtracted out.

Suppose that Linda has $5450 in annual medical expenses. Three percent of her $15,000 income is $450. Anything beyond that—in this case $5000—can be subtracted from income to find adjusted income. Thus, her adjusted income is $10,000.

Thirty percent of $10,000 is $3000, so she can get an apartment for $3000/year, which is $250/month.

At Bradshaw Senior Community, the income limits are $24,240 for one person and $27,720 for two. The rent calculations are done a little differently and also vary with apartment size. In some cases, rents as a percentage of income could be higher than at the other two sites.

Calculations for all three sites are complex and waiting lists are common, so it is reasonable to start checking out this option and get help with the calculations to see if you qualify well before you think that you might want to make such a move.

Applicants for HUD apartments need to provide documentation of their income and assets initially as part of the application process and annually after that, to show that they are eligible for this housing.

Appealing features of these HUD-subsidized complexes are discussed in the next article. Two subsequent articles will describe an Arizona state program that can provide subsidized housing and medical care for life for some people who have lived in Arizona for a very long time.

22

Subsidized Housing:
The Experience

The previous column discussed costs of HUD-subsidized senior apartments. This article describes features of three: Casa de Pinos (run by Retirement Housing Foundation, affiliated with the United Church of Christ), Village Tower (run by the Evangelical Lutheran Good Samaritan Society), and Bradshaw Senior Community.

The sites appear clean, quiet, and well managed. Some features clearly reflect financial constraints—kitchen cabinets are more likely to be made of plywood than of, say, cherry hardwood, for example.

That said, the apartments appear very functional. For example, two-bedroom apartments in Village Tower feature—astonishingly—six large closets.

Bradshaw is the newest site, and its physical plant is very attractive.

The two faith-based nonprofits provide a wide array of extra services and support, and work hard to create a sense of community.

Casa de Pinos manager Dena Maiolo said, "Our mission is to provide quality, affordable housing for the elderly that allows them to live independently as long as possible." Many residents don't have family in their lives, and fellow residents watch out for each other.

Staff members provide surprisingly personalized help. For example, Marla Tibbits, the manager at Village Tower, noted, "I get calls from residents' children saying, 'My mom's phone has been busy for the last three hours. Could you see if she left it off the hook?' Or a resident may say, 'I haven't seen so-and-so for a few days. Will you check to make sure she's okay?'"

In mid-December, Casa de Pinos manager Maiolo and social service coordinator Dee Blaschke described their plans to personally cook Christmas brunch for the residents and to distribute gifts provided through the "Be a Santa to a Senior" program organized by the senior care organization Home Instead.

HUD provides rent subsidies, but services depend on donations and volunteers. Social service coordinators at the two nonprofits help residents get free or low-cost help with housecleaning, buying groceries, fixing meals, doing laundry, driving to doctors' appointments, etc.

Volunteer organizations such as People Who Care play important roles. Meals on Wheels is a major presence.

Staff members identify issues and also coordinate with family. For example, Casa de Pinos asked the Area Agency on Aging, part of NACOG (Northern Arizona Council of Governments), to evaluate a resident who was struggling, and then located needed services.

Bradshaw Senior Community operates more like a standard apartment complex, without a social service coordinator or extensive extra services.

Typical features at all three sites include libraries, television, monthly birthday celebrations, potluck dinners, seasonal activities such as caroling and Thanksgiving and Christmas parties, emergency pull cords, coin-operated laundries, and activity rooms with pianos, kitchens, jigsaw puzzles and games.

Small, well-behaved pets are welcome.

Typically, residents may reserve a kitchen/activity room for family gatherings.

Bradshaw Senior Community and Village Tower each have a pool table and exercise equipment. Bradshaw sports a theatre room, computer access, and movies, and receives donations from Costco of day-old bread and muffins for residents.

Casa de Pinos mentioned Walmart, Costco, and Safeway as major donors.

At Village Tower, one may find a drawing class, music, and bingo; Wii bowling, complete with a multi-site annual competition and a huge trophy; a beauty salon;

Books on Wheels—and a magnifying machine to make reading possible for people with limited eyesight; and regular transportation to grocery stores, Wal-Mart, and the mall. (While a $2 donation is suggested for transportation, no one is ever refused a ride for not contributing.)

Village Tower plans to offer free Wi-Fi to residents by the end of 2013. The maintenance man delivers monthly food boxes from an outside agency to eligible residents; anything they don't want goes to a common area for other residents.

At Casa de Pinos, residents can get free greeting cards, and a recent monthly newsletter included a homemade word search puzzle containing all residents' names.

When asked what she liked best about living at Casa de Pinos, one resident immediately replied, "The freedom, and the people."

While HUD-subsidized apartments—particularly the older ones—are not as fancy as those in upscale retirement communities, residents' quality of life and satisfaction may be quite similar.

23

Arizona Pioneers' Home:
What Is It?

A stately brick building overlooking the city from the top of a hill just south of downtown is the Arizona Pioneers' Home. For long-time Arizona residents in good health but of limited means who are seeking a new place to live, it can provide a satisfying alternative to other options for senior housing and care.

It has space for about 155 residents and currently houses less than one hundred.

Established by statute more than a hundred years ago—when Arizona was still a territory—the Pioneers' Home is an unusual institution.

Created to provide housing and care for people who contributed to Arizona's development and who don't have a lot of money, it generally accepts only residents who have lived in Arizona for at least fifty years and who are over the age of seventy.

When they enter, residents must be able to walk and to manage without assistance typical activities of daily living such as dressing, bathing, eating and so forth. They do not need to be able to prepare food, as all meals and snacks are provided, and their accommodations do not include individual kitchens.

If their health deteriorates after they have become residents, in almost all cases the Pioneers' Home will continue to take care of them for the rest of their lives.

It also offers cemetery plots in its own cemetery, at no charge to residents.

A few residents enter the Arizona Pioneers' Home under a disabled miners program, for Arizona miners who are either poor or whose health was damaged by their work in Arizona mines.

Those applicants need be only sixty years old, and they may enter with health issues. Disabled miners are not required to pay anything for their housing or standard care.

Residents are not charged any kind of admission fee or up-front lump sum when they move in, although such charges are common in other communities that commit to providing life-long housing and medical care.

Residents are required to have Medicare coverage and to maintain a Medigap policy to help with medical expenses not covered by Medicare.

Pioneers, as residents other than miners are termed, must reimburse the state for as much of the cost of their care, currently $4702/month, as they can. Residents may keep enough money to pay the premiums on their Medigap policies, and they may keep another $200/month for personal expenses.

Someone with income (after subtracting the cost of a Medigap policy) of $250/month would keep $200 and pay just $50. Someone with total income of $20,000 a month would pay $4702.

However, people who can afford to pay a significant portion of the full amount—more than $56,000 a year—are likely to consider other options. For example, the base rate for assisted living in an apartment at Granite Gate with about four times the space is roughly $30,000 a year.

The state ends up contributing about $5 million a year to the operation of the Pioneers' Home, and about another $1 million comes from its residents.

Applicants are encouraged to have all known medical, dental, and eye care needs addressed before they move in. The Pioneers' Home typically will not cover pre-existing conditions unless Medicare pays for them.

How do residents pay for care that is not covered, when they can typically keep only $200/month in income? In some cases their children may provide the money, or they may draw on their own financial reserves.

Unlike the case with Medicaid, residents are not required to spend down their assets to be eligible to move in to the Arizona Pioneers' Home.

For example, if they have investments totaling $100,000 that pay dividends of $3000 a year, that income averages out to $250/month and that $250 would be counted in their monthly income.

However, they are not required to turn in the $100,000 in assets in this example. They may keep or use that money as they like, whether it is for medical care, travel, clothing, or whatever else they choose.

The next column will describe the accommodations and other features of the Arizona Pioneers' Home.

24

Arizona Pioneers' Home: The Experience

Like a favorite elderly relative, the Arizona Pioneers' Home is quirky but engaging. Every comment I've heard about the place reflects great respect bordering on reverence.

Home to roughly one hundred Pioneers—elderly long-term residents of Arizona, typically with limited means—and disabled miners, the Arizona Pioneers' Home has a unique approach to creating a pleasant environment.

All new residents move into double-occupancy rooms, and are on probation for sixty days. If they don't get along well with the staff and other residents during that period, they are asked to leave.

Superintendent Ted Ihrman remarked, "We may not all be one big happy family, but we are something very close to it!"

Housing is akin to dorm rooms or hospital rooms, rather than apartments. Generally, residents have about 144 square feet each—roughly 12 feet x 12 feet. The ability to get along with others is highly prized partly because everyone lives in such close quarters.

A single bathroom may be shared by two rooms—four people—or may even be down the hall. Each person may have only a few feet of closet space.

Other characteristics also seem reminiscent of summer camp or a boarding school of the 1950s. For example, the Pioneers' Home does not have a health center or medical center or nursing wing or doctor's office—it has "infirmaries."

When asked about this choice of terms, Ihrman started laughing. "The state of Arizona told us, as part of an inspection a few years ago, that we should change the name. We took it to the residents, and they said, 'They've been infirmaries for a hundred years! Why change now?' So we didn't."

The Pioneers' Home operates with more staff, and higher skill levels of staffing, than is typical in other retirement communities with a similar population. For example, at least one registered nurse is on duty 24/7.

Because the Pioneers' Home operates under its own set of state statutes, the Arizona Department of Health Services inspects the site but doesn't post the results as it does for sites that it licenses.

Residents with whom I spoke were uniformly friendly and articulate. When asked what they liked best, typical answers included, "The people and the way they get along together," "It's a good place to be," "They treat you well," and "The security—knowing that I'll be taken care of."

When asked what they'd change, answers ranged from "Nothing," offered after a long, thoughtful pause, to "Give everyone a private room," although in that case the speaker went on to say that of course it was necessary to trade off that luxury against the benefit of being able to take care of more people.

The Pioneers' Home provides amenities such as a library, a computer, Wi-Fi access, monthly birthday parties, card games, bingo, and transportation to stores.

A recent outing took residents to the Verde Valley Archeology Center. Other outings may see residents at the rodeo or the county fair, fishing, gold panning, visiting museums, and taking in community performances.

A recent calendar listed groups/events such as a writing and poetry class, a walking club, a sing-along, crafts, a variety of religious services, and a visit from the Presbyterian Singers.

Arizona Pioneers' Home also boasts its own rhythm band, concerts by resident musicians, and weekly bowling—in the lobby!

V

In-Home Services

An alternative to moving is to stay in your home and have services come to you.

25

Discover
What In-Home Services Are Needed

Previous articles have discussed housing and care options that involve moving out of the home that you—or an aging relative—may have lived in for many years. What if you or they don't want to move?

If you or an aging relative needs a service, the odds are good that other people do, too—and that someone has set up a business or a nonprofit to meet the need.

In the Prescott area, dozens—if not hundreds—of for-profit and not-for-profit organizations are ready to help manage life at home.

A resource directory at www.seniorconnection.us lists service providers in 33 categories such as "in-home—medical" (16 organizations), "in-home—non-medical" (44 organizations), and "personal services" (15 organizations).

That last category even includes one business, Mobile Haircutting Services, whose owner KC Cain will come to your home to cut your hair and provide other salon-type services such as manicures and pedicures.

But where do you even start? A good first step is to arrange for a comprehensive assessment by a Geriatric Care Manager certified by the National Association of Professional Geriatric Care Managers.

Certified Geriatric Care Managers meet extensive requirements for education, supervised professional experience after earning one or more degrees, and proficiency exams leading to certification.

These qualifications help ensure that they understand and can effectively address a broad array of issues facing the elderly.

Ron Goldman is a Certified Geriatric Care Manager (and Licensed Master of Social Work as well as a Licensed Fiduciary) who founded Arizona Elder Care LLC (www.ArizonaElderCare.com).

He explained that a comprehensive assessment typically starts with three to four hours spent with the individual or couple in their home to understand the specifics of their situation.

This time may be split into two or three sessions if necessary. Then the care manager prepares a report detailing the current status of the individual(s), services needed, and options for getting those services. The report also identifies probable future needs as well.

The care manager will meet with the individual(s) and family members as appropriate to discuss findings, conclusions and recommendations.

The Area Agency on Aging of the Northern Arizona Council of Governments (NACOG) also offers needs assessments under its case management program, for people age 60-plus.

The agency prioritizes providing services to people who are frailer and older, and who have lower income. Call toll-free (877) 521-3500 for information and referrals.

Why not just get a free assessment from any of the many agencies that provide in-home services?

You may find that a free assessment serves simply to identify useful in-home services that the organization doing the assessment offers. You might not immediately realize that a number of other services that the organization *doesn't* offer are needed as well.

Issues that you or your relative may be facing may include the risk of financial mismanagement, dangers of complications and side effects associated with taking a large number of prescription drugs, safety problems arising from living in a cluttered environment, potential emotional concerns such as depression and social isolation, possible health problems resulting from keeping or eating spoiled food, risks of falls related to poor balance, malnutrition if buying food and preparing meals have become difficult, specific concerns related to particular medical conditions, and so forth.

A Certified Geriatric Care Manager can help you understand the different types of service organizations, which services each offers, and the pros and cons of using each.

The value of this independent perspective was emphasized when a reader wrote to me about her confusion arising from the fact that two different organizations each said that it was the only provider in the area that could deliver a certain type of service.

In fact, seven organizations in town are licensed to provide that particular service—and one of the two that claimed to her that it is "the only one" isn't even licensed to provide that service at all.

26

Qualify For
Home Health Services

If you want to stay in your home but have medical conditions that make caring for yourself tricky, what services can help you?

Available services fall into three major buckets: medical services, "para-medical" services, and non-medical services. This article focuses on medical services, also known as home health services.

This article assumes that the individual who needs in-home care is age 65-plus and is enrolled in Medicare, the federal health insurance program for the elderly and disabled.

Home health services are covered at no cost to enrollees in traditional Medicare if four conditions are met.

The first is that the individual is homebound. Interesting, "homebound" doesn't mean that the person never leaves home. Medicare explains its definition:

"Leaving your home isn't recommended because of your condition. Your condition keeps you from leaving home without help (such as using a wheelchair or walker, needing special transportation, or getting help from another person). Leaving home takes a considerable and taxing effort.

"A person may leave home for medical treatment or short, infrequent absences for non-medical reasons, such as attending religious services. You can still get home health care if you attend adult day care, but you would get the home care services in your home."

The second condition is that you are under a doctor's care, and that the doctor has created and regularly updates a plan of care for you.

The third is that your doctor certifies that you need physical therapy, occupational therapy, speech therapy, medical social services and/or "intermittent" skilled nursing care (meaning that you don't need skilled nursing all—or even most of—the hours in a day).

Generally, the care must be medically necessary and recognized as appropriate for the individual's condition. It must require a skilled caregiver to deliver it.

Medicare will even pay for help with bathing, dressing, etc. if the doctor certifies your need—but only if you are getting other higher-skilled services such as skilled nursing care as well.

The fourth condition is that the care must be provided by a home health agency that is Medicare-certified.

Explanations follow for some of Medicare's terms.

"Examples of skilled nursing care include: giving IV drugs, shots, or tube feedings; changing dressings; and teaching about prescription drugs or diabetes care. Any service that could be done safely by a non-medical person (or by yourself) without the supervision of a nurse, **isn't** skilled nursing care." (emphasis in the original)

Medicare doesn't cover full-time skilled nursing care, and it draws the line well before 24/7. For example, if you need care more than eight hours a day seven days a week, Medicare will not pay.

Medicare defines physical therapy as "treatment of injury and disease by mechanical means, such as heat, light, exercise, and massage."

Occupational therapy, contrary to popular belief, does not necessarily have anything to do with performing a job for pay. Medicare defines it as "services given to help you return to usual activities (such as bathing, preparing meals, and housekeeping) after illness either on an inpatient or outpatient basis."

Speech therapy addresses issues not only with speaking but also with swallowing.

Medical social services "help you with social and emotional concerns related to your illness. This might include counseling or help in finding resources in your community."

Medical supplies are also covered if they are "essential items that the home health team uses to conduct home visits or to carry out services the physician has ordered to treat or diagnose a patient's illness or injury. . . The home health agency provides these supplies for their use with the patient."

Personal care, or "home health aide services" assist you with "daily living activities," generally considered to be bathing, dressing, using the toilet, eating, moving from one place to another (e.g., bed to chair), and walking.

Most commonly, services are provided for perhaps an hour or two a few times a week.

Medicare explains its requirements and what home health services are covered in a brochure available at http://www.medicare.gov/Pubs/pdf/10969.pdf.

Medicare defines many of its terms in a glossary at http://www.medicare.gov/Homehealthcompare/Resources/Glossary.aspx.

The next column discusses home health agencies.

27

Choose an Agency
To Provide Home Health Services

The previous article described medical services available at home, possibly creating an alternative to living in an assisted living center or skilled nursing facility. But how do you choose an agency that will provide the quality of care you or your relatives need?

Recommendations from doctors, nurses, family and friends are a good place to start.

A second source of information is Medicare. Services to Medicare enrollees need to be provided by Medicare-certified agencies if Medicare is to pay, and Medicare collects and posts a great deal of information about each agency at its Home Health Compare website at http://www.medicare.gov/homehealthcompare/.

A recent search for providers that offer services in Prescott yielded a list of seven agencies. The site has a "compare" feature that allows you to choose up to three organizations to compare at once.

The site lists the percentage of time that each agency met certain objectives, and how those numbers compare to Arizona and national averages.

For example, 75 percent of Granite Mountain Home Care's patients who were having trouble breathing when they started getting care had less trouble breathing when they finished getting care. The national average is 64 percent, so one can conclude that this agency is doing a good job in this area.

Good Samaritan Society Prescott Home Health checks whether patients have had pneumonia shots 94 percent of the time; the national average is 68 percent, so clearly Good Samaritan pays much more attention to this issue than is typical.

As another example, 89 percent of Granite Mountain Home Care's patients would recommend the agency to friends and family; the Arizona average is 72 percent, so Granite Mountain is outperforming the average by quite a large margin.

The website identifies 27 measures, and an agency that does a good job on one measure may not do a good job on some others. You may want to look at all the measures, paying particular attention to ones relevant to your care or the care of your friend or relative.

For example, a measure related to care of people with diabetes might mean little for people who don't have that condition. A measure concerned with wound healing after surgery isn't of much interest for people who haven't had, and don't contemplate having, surgery.

Medicare suggests a number of questions to ask when choosing a home health agency. It makes sense to talk with two or three agencies before choosing one. Asking thoughtful questions and taking careful notes can help you get the most out of this little-understood benefit.

The brochure "Medicare and Home Health Care" found at http://www.medicare.gov/Pubs/pdf/10969.pdf offers a checklist to help you choose an agency.

A few questions it suggests are:

- Can the agency meet my special needs for language or cultural preferences?
- Does the agency have the staff to provide the services I need, or can it help me arrange for additional services I may need, such as Meals on Wheels?
- Does the agency have staff available at night and on weekends for emergencies?

AARP offers another, and in places more extensive, home health agency checklist of its own, available at http://assets.aarp.org/external_sites/caregiving/checklists/checklist_inHomeCare.html.

It is worth noting that Medicare will pay for services for any individual from only one home health agency at a time. You can switch agencies at any time, but it won't pay two agencies if you are receiving services from two at the same time.

According to Allison Kantor, Home Health Clinical Supervisor at Good Samaritan, most people don't realize two important facts about Medicare coverage of home health services: first, Medicare typically pays 100 percent of the cost, assuming that people have not assigned their Medicare benefits to an HMO.

Second, while Medicare will typically cover a maximum of only 100 days of care in a skilled nursing facility after a hospital stay, there is no time limit for coverage of home health services.

Kantor noted that sometimes people pay out-of-pocket for home health services that Medicare doesn't cover, to reduce disruption for the patient. For example, she explained, "They may hire us to come to the house to draw blood instead of taking Grandma to the lab."

28

See What Non-Medical In-Home Services Are Available

Suppose that you or elderly relatives find the logistics of daily living to be a bit overwhelming.

Imagine needing help with any or all of the following, or similar activities: setting up a pillbox with medicines to take at different times of day for the coming week; shopping for groceries; preparing meals; keeping track of and disposing of food that is expiring or spoiled; walking the dog; doing dishes; changing the sheets, caring for houseplants; remembering to pay bills; going on outings to concerts, church services, or other events; remembering and getting to doctors' appointments, and keeping track of follow-ups afterwards; dealing with a feeding tube; and/or bathing and dressing.

Often, people either don't have family members available, or prefer to address their needs without calling on family, and so turn to service agencies for help.

How many different agencies would it take to get all of the above needs addressed? Five or ten? The good news is that the answer is probably one or two.

Many agencies can help with non-medical services such as shopping, cleaning, and transportation, and several options are even available for handling services that fall between those activities and care that requires highly trained professionals such as registered nurses.

Marsha Douglas, the Area Supervisor for Abrio Care, explained that the agency has staff trained to handle what it terms "para-medical" services, such as helping with colostomy bags, urinary catheters, and feeding tubes; checking oxygen saturation levels and blood pressure; and setting up pill boxes for the coming week.

Some agencies can help with the transition from one level or location of care to another.

For example, when people come home after a hospital stay, they are often unclear about what medicines they are supposed to continue taking and what follow-ups need to occur, and their health can suffer as a result.

Douglas noted that Abrio Care offers a service called Discharge Express that includes activities such as transporting people home after hospitalization, picking up new medicines, checking their home for safety, preparing a meal, tucking them into bed and returning the next day to ensure that they are doing well.

Mary Mackenzie, Administrator and Director of Nursing for Granite Mountain Home Care and Hospice, noted that when patients transition from its home health services (skilled medical care) to non-medical services provided by its Granite Mountain Private Duty arm, it coordinates care to ensure that the transition is a safe and smooth one for its clients.

Abrio and Granite Mountain are among the agencies that can handle virtually all of the non-medical tasks and activities listed at the beginning of this article, as well as many not listed.

The non-medical home care agency Home Instead lists many activities that its caregivers are prepared to handle, including some that you might not expect: assisting with entertaining, reminiscing about the past, writing letters, and discussing current events.

Non-medical agencies may provide services a few hours a week, or in eight-hour shifts, or around the clock seven days a week.

They typically try hard to create a good fit between clients and caregivers based on the client's specific needs.

Douglas of Abrio noted, "Studies show that 85 percent of people want to stay at home," rather than move into an assisted living or skilled nursing facility, and Abrio works hard to help them safely continue to meet this goal.

Agencies that help people with activities of daily living such as bathing, dressing, using the toilet, and so forth may get paid by a variety of sources such as the Veterans Administration, Arizona Medicaid (ALTCS),

Arizona Department of Developmental Disabilities, the Area Agency on Aging of the Northern Arizona Council of Governments, long-term care insurance, and people receiving the services or their relatives.

Mackenzie of Granite Mountain noted that people are often covered by Medicare for home health services (skilled care) and after two to four months they may transition to non-medical care that may be covered by Medicaid (ALTCS).

Typical charges for people paying privately are roughly $18-19/hour.

The next column will discuss how agencies screen and supervise people who work with vulnerable adults.

29

Know How Agencies Screen and Supervise Employees in Your Home

If you want to stay in your home but need help with some of the details—getting ready for the day in the mornings, running errands, and so forth—you may decide to engage an agency that provides in-home non-medical services.

But how do you know that a stranger in your home won't take advantage of you?

Marsha Douglas, Area Supervisor for Abrio Care and Felice Neely, Staffing Supervisor of Granite Mountain's Private Duty (non-medical home services) arm, explained some of their safeguards to me.

Both agencies undertake at least three extensive background checks of all applicants, one of which in both cases draws on a federal database. Other checks may involve steps such as searching a private national database for criminal activities, and reviewing driving records provided by a third party (not by the applicant).

Caregivers must also obtain a fingerprint clearance card, which indicates that the state has cleared the applicant to work with vulnerable populations.

Abrio also requires caregivers to undergo more than 50 hours of training and pass a two- to three-hour combined written and hands-on exam at the end to complete Arizona's Direct Care Worker training program. The course covers legal and ethical responsibilities as well as dozens of other topics.

Both agencies hire only people with at least a year's experience, and routinely provide additional training, including specialized training at the client's home when a client requires specific special services.

Neely noted that when Granite Mountain caregivers arrive at and leave a client's home, they must call in to an automated system from the client's landline or cell phone. These calls help ensure that clients are billed only for time that caregivers spend on-site and that caregivers do not work unauthorized hours.

Douglas of Abrio Care and Mary Mackenzie, the Administrator and Director of Nursing at Granite Mountain's Home Care and Hospice arm (which is closely integrated with its non-medical home services arm), both noted that caregivers keep a log book in the home reporting on the client's status and activities during every visit, available to supervisors and to family members.

Further, supervisors routinely visit the client's home to help ensure that everything is in order.

Granite Mountain is implementing a new system that will allow authorized family members to access a password-protected website to get information about caregiver visits and their relative's status.

How are clients' finances protected? Neely and Douglas both described similar extensive and detailed controls. A meeting is held with each new client to discuss how money will be handled if caregivers are expected to run errands.

Caregivers are not allowed access to a client's standard debit or credit cards or checkbooks. A client may provide a prepaid card with a fixed limit, or a signed check if all the information is filled in.

Both Abrio and Granite Mountain ask that caregivers not be given cash for purchases, and require that caregivers give to the client all receipts documenting purchases with prepaid cards or checks.

Both agencies also require new employees to sign documents that prohibit them from becoming signers on clients' checking accounts or becoming powers of attorney for clients. They may not be involved in changing clients' wills or become beneficiaries in clients' wills.

Douglas of Abrio noted that employees are forbidden from taking anything at all from clients—cash, Christmas presents, anything. If they do, they will lose their jobs as soon as the situation is discovered.

At Granite Mountain, employees are not permitted to work for a Granite Mountain client outside of the Granite Mountain contract, and must not work directly for a client within a year of leaving Granite Mountain.

Both agencies report that the safeguards they have in place have protected clients to date.

Neely noted, "We would cover any client losses that resulted from any employee misconduct."

Douglas of Abrio noted, "Where people get into trouble is hiring people off the street, without the training, supervision, and safeguards that major agencies put in place."

Don't hesitate to ask any agency you are considering how it safeguards its clients.

VI

Senior Move Managers
Can Help

You don't need to delay a move to a retirement community because you don't know what to do with all your "stuff" or how you'll get along with less space. Help is available.

Experts can also help improve safety and convenience in your home if you decide not to move.

30

Deal With
a Lifetime's Possessions

Perhaps you are considering moving to a retirement community, but when you look at the house you've lived in for 10 or 20 or 40 years, you feel discouraged. You remember how hard it was to organize and pack everything the last time you moved—and that may have been decades ago.

You have a sneaking suspicion that you just can't get there from here, and even though you'd like to move and enjoy life without all the work involved in keeping a house, you start to think that your executor will be the one who will finally figure out what to do with your high school yearbooks, 5-1/4" floppy disks from your first computer, 40 years of tax returns, shoeboxes of photos, the suitcase that's perfectly good except for one broken zipper, clothes you haven't worn since Bill Clinton was president, old VCRs and cell phones, and the always growing pile of mystery keys in the junk drawer.

You remember wistfully your favorite quotation from Henry David Thoreau in high school: "A man is rich in proportion to the number of things which he can afford to let alone." Somehow, you have strayed from that idea.

You vaguely realize that you might be moving from, say, a 2500-square-foot house into perhaps an 800-square-foot apartment. Is there any hope? Absolutely!

Enter the "Senior Move Manager," a member of the National Association of Senior Move Managers (NASMM).

According to its website, "A Senior Move Manager is a professional who specializes in assisting older adults and their families with the emotional and physical aspects of relocation and/or 'aging in place'. . . Senior Move Managers guide clients through a journey that's often as much about sorting through a lifetime's worth of memories as it is about possessions."

See the NASMM website at www.nasmm.org for more information and for a free brochure called "Your Guide to Stress-Free Rightsizing and Relocation."

At one end of the spectrum, Senior Move Managers may simply work with an individual or couple to develop a customized master plan for their move. Individuals and family members then perform the tasks indicated.

At the other end of the spectrum, a Senior Move Manager may personally perform or arrange for the performance of every single task, such as deciding what to keep, giving away or selling the rest, packing, moving, unpacking—and even hanging pictures in the new home, preparing the vacated house for sale, and selecting a Realtor.

Barbara Kult, the owner of In Your Space Consulting (www.inyourspaceaz.com), is a Senior Move Manager who serves north and central Arizona, including the Prescott area. She can help people move to and from other parts of the country as well.

She explained that when someone hires her, she starts by asking a series of questions that helps her clients clarify what is important to them.

She also obtains floor plans of the home that they will be moving into, typically an independent living or assisted living apartment, or even a room in a long-term care (nursing) or hospice facility.

With this information, she can help her clients visualize how their belongings will fit in their new home, and can provide guidance as she helps them to sort through their belongings to decide what to keep and what to let go.

She commented, "I do all the physical work. I try to involve clients as much as possible in the decision-making," although about a quarter of the time, she is hired by an adult child who is making arrangements to move a parent with dementia or another illness, and the person moving may have a limited ability to make decisions.

In these cases, she works closely with both people to get the best results possible for the person moving.

Kult noted, "Through careful planning and compassion, we have only had positive experiences for my clients and for me. I really love what I do. It is very gratifying. I respectfully enter people's lives to help them at a challenging time. I try to meet people where they are."

Next week's column will go into more detail about the senior move process.

31

Create a "Blueprint for Success" for the Move

A quick quiz—which of these would you prefer to do:

- Listen to fingernails on a chalkboard for hours and hours every day?
- Figure out how to downsize to move from your four-bedroom house to a one-bedroom apartment in a retirement community?

While many people might be tempted to choose the fingernails-on-a-chalkboard alternative, it doesn't have to be that way. Last week's column described a service provided by experts called Senior Move Managers who help people move from their homes of many years to more manageable apartments—and who can help make the move a positive experience.

Barbara Kult, the owner of In Your Space Consulting, is a Senior Move Manager certified through the National Association of Senior Move Managers. She can help with moves to, from and within north and central Arizona, including Prescott.

Once she understands what matters most to her clients and the space they will be moving into, she explained, "I work with them on developing their 'Wish List'—if they could take whatever they want, what would it be?"

She creates a floor plan with them showing where their belongings will go. Clients see that "they CAN take many treasured items. This plan becomes the blueprint for success."

Next, she said, "After looking at what will fit, we look at everything that's left. We [may] do estate sales. . . to help offset some of their moving costs."

If family members want any items that the elderly person is not planning to keep, "We encourage them to gift them." However, when family members realize that they will need to pay for shipping, which can be expensive, "They may decide, 'Oh, I don't really want that anyway.'"

Sometimes people have been hanging on to belongings because it seems a waste to throw them away, or because they feel obligated to keep them. In these cases, the Senior Move Manager helps work through the emotional issues.

In some cases, a Senior Move Manager may recommend or arrange for old pictures and other documents to be digitized—scanned, for example; old home movies might be turned into CDs.

"A lot of my clients are computer-savvy," Kult noted, and they can scan and organize electronic files themselves. Sensitive documents no longer needed may be shredded.

Kult explained, "The ideal client says, 'I am going to move in a year,' and then at six months gets really serious. The biggest drawback that I find is that people wait too long in life to make that move, and it just gets harder and harder. Then it becomes a crisis move—everything in one week's time."

She noted, "The typical mistake is that people think that they can do it themselves. They get started, they've committed to a move date, but they're not ready—they aren't asking for help soon enough. They may feel overwhelmed. A lot of people say, 'My family will help me,' but then there are conflicts. We step in as needed. Senior Move Managers are trained to understand the emotional component of a move—it's at least 50 percent of the picture."

Sometimes, Kult noted, planned tasks need to be set aside for the moment in order to address the emotional issues.

Kult described a couple who gradually—over nine months—implemented the plan that she had created with them. As she worked with them at each visit to sort and donate belongings, they said, "Oh, my gosh, we feel so much lighter!"

At the end of the project, they said that they had enjoyed that nine months in their decluttered house more than all the previous years.

Kult finds that most clients describe similar feelings. They may have felt weighed down for years by belongings that were no longer of much use to them but which they had trouble letting go.

She is typically able to help them make decisions they are happy with about which belongings are enriching their lives and which ones no longer fill a need. They often feel that a great burden has been lifted when the less important belongings are gone.

32

Reduce Clutter To Age In Place Safely

The previous two weeks' columns discussed "senior move management," a process that helps people make the transition from a house they may have lived in for many years to a smaller home, typically an apartment in a retirement community.

What if you plan to stay in your home for a while longer, but sort of wish that you were moving, just so that you could start over without the accumulated weight of a lifetime of possessions?

You can engage the same experts that help people move. Despite the name, Senior Move Managers such as Barbara Kult of In Your Space Consulting (www.inyourspaceaz.com) also offer decluttering and aging-in-place services.

Kult helps clients identify how they use each room in their home, what health conditions they are dealing with, and what's important to them. She creates a floor plan showing details of each room.

In a key step early in the process, she uses an extensive safety checklist to identify any hazards that the individual or couple faces at home.

For example, if the client uses a cane, walker, or wheelchair, Kult may propose rearranging or replacing furniture so that the individual can safely maneuver around the house without catching any assistive devices on protruding furniture.

She may recommend eliminating furniture with sharp corners, or rickety chairs or tables that always seem to be on the verge of tipping over. If rugs pose a trip hazard, she will suggest either fastening them securely or removing them.

Chemicals and other hazardous substances that are expired or no longer needed can be sorted and properly disposed of. Examples include old medicines, paint, and cleaning products. Basements and garages often contain a bewildering array of leftover toxic materials.

Once Kult understands how clients use their homes and what safety hazards need to be addressed, she begins working with them to identify other changes that can allow them to age in place more comfortably and safely.

She can help them eliminate 25-75 percent of the belongings and papers that have accumulated over the years but that no longer serve a purpose, including clothing that they no longer use. "The reality is that the average person uses 20 percent of what they own; the other 80 percent is fluff and stuff," Kult explained.

She helps clients distinguish between cherished belongings and less important items.

Another key step is to make needed belongings easier to access. Simple modifications to closets can put needed items within reach, and custom-designed rollout shelves in kitchens and bathrooms allow belongings in the back to be seen, reached, and used.

Targeted improvements can create what Kult terms "layered lighting." Just as it is often helpful to dress in layers that can be added or subtracted as needed, a variety of lighting fixtures can be put in place to augment natural light with different types and levels of lighting as needed.

Stairways may be made safer by adding inexpensive improvements such as handrails, friction strips, or reflective tape. Handrails might also be installed in bathrooms.

In some cases, more extensive changes might be proposed, such as adding a riding chair lift to a stairway or replacing a bath tub with a walk-in or roll-in shower.

At times, a Senior Move Manager might recommend remote sensing technology.

For example, sensors that detect motion might be placed in the kitchen. If the resident hasn't entered the kitchen by noon, for instance, an alert might be sent to an adult child, who could call to ask if her parent is okay.

A variant on remote sensing is a waterproof pendant that the resident can wear, with a button to press if she falls or experiences another emergency and can't get to a phone.

In most cases, such devices work like OnStar for cars: a live operator responds and dispatches whatever emergency services are needed. Sophisticated devices can even detect when the wearer has fallen, and summon help automatically.

Through a combination of decluttering and aging-in-place services, older adults can get many of the benefits of moving to a safer and more streamlined home without ever actually leaving their house.

VII

Prevent Medical Problems in Assisted Living and Long-Term Care

Contrary to popular belief, it's necessary to pay attention to ensure that needed care is received and unwanted care is not—even if you or your loved ones are living at sites that generally provide excellent care.

33

Watch For Overdoses

Suppose that you have helped an elderly relative move into an assisted living apartment or into a room in a nursing or skilled nursing facility. Now you can breathe a big sigh of relief, knowing that they will be well taken care of, right?

Not so fast.

It is true that the employees in many well run assisted living and nursing/skilled nursing facilities are well trained, well intentioned, skilled, caring, compassionate individuals. You may discover that they even have more patience with your elderly relative than you do.

It is still possible for major errors and gaps in care to arise—and you, who may not even have any training in health care, may be the first one to notice.

This article and several more will discuss this issue.

Lisa observed that her father, who had recently moved into a high-quality assisted living facility, had become very lethargic. She wondered if he was getting too high a dose of a newly prescribed anti-anxiety medicine.

She discovered that the American Geriatrics Society has useful reference guides at www.americangeriatrics.org under the heading, "AGS Updated Beers Criteria for Potentially Inappropriate Medication Use in Older Adults (2012)." Clicking on the link calls up a whole list of available downloads.

Under the heading "Public Education Resources," some of the titles are: "AGS Beers Criteria Summary—For Patients & Caregivers," "10 Medications Older Adults Should Avoid," and "What to Do and What to Ask Your Healthcare Provider if a Medication You Take is Listed in the Beers Criteria."

Lisa found these all useful. The first and second both revealed that the drug her father was taking is known to cause problems in the elderly. She also consulted the "Beers Criteria Pocket Card" listed under "Clinical Tools." While intended for doctors and other health care professionals, it was also helpful to her.

She met with her father's doctor. She used the information she had learned.

For example, asking questions rather than assuming that the doctor has done something wrong is almost certain to get better results.

Possible questions include, "What is this drug being prescribed for?" "Are new symptoms that have recently surfaced possible side effects of this drug?" "Is there a safer alternative that might be tried?"

Lisa also asked if the dose could be reduced, and if a plan could be created to wean her father off the drug. The doctor agreed to reduce the dosage immediately by one-third.

Lisa discussed this change with the staff at the assisted living facility so that they would know that the prescription was changing and not be surprised by that.

Over the next several weeks, she did not see any improvement in her father's condition. In fact, he seemed more lethargic than before.

About a month later, she received the usual monthly bill from the assisted living center. She found multiple charges for the drug, and discovered that one pharmacy had filled a prescription for the original dose on January 31, and a second pharmacy had filled a prescription for the reduced dose on February 01.

Because two pharmacies were used, neither pharmacist—nor their computer systems—saw both prescriptions.

Lisa discovered that her father had been given both doses every day in February—meaning that he got two-and-a-half times the amount he was intended to get at that point.

It is not clear exactly what went wrong. Perhaps the first prescription was set up to refill automatically, which is a common arrangement, with drugs being sent and billed to the assisted living center.

Perhaps it simply didn't occur to the doctor that he needed to cancel that original order.

Had Lisa's father been living independently, that minor oversight might not have caused any problems, because most people would not pick up and pay for two prescriptions for the same drug just a day apart.

However, in assisted living or nursing facilities, staff may not question the doctor's orders, and elderly patients never even see pill bottles. Instead they are simply handed a little cup with some pills in it and told, "Swallow these!"

Lisa's experience highlights this reality: it is necessary to follow up to ensure that expected changes happen as intended.

34

Check For Care Omissions

The previous article discussed how duplicate prescriptions might arise, overdosing your loved one who lives in assisted living or nursing/skilled nursing. This article discusses the opposite problem: how needed care may be omitted.

Isabel's mother Gretchen has been living in a skilled nursing facility in Boston for nearly six years. When Isabel lived nearby, she visited Gretchen at least once a month. Now living in California, Isabel stays in regular contact with the facility by phone and email.

She just visited in person for the first time in ten months. When she arrived, she spent a couple hours reading her mother's chart, her right as her mother's authorized health care representative.

She suddenly realized that a recent summary of her mother's condition made no mention of the osteoporosis her mother had had for the last 30 years—and no mention of the drug she was supposed to be taking for it, either.

She felt like Sherlock Holmes, in the case where the important fact was that the dog did NOT bark in the night.

She pointed out the omission of osteoporosis to a nurse, and a couple days later the nurse told her, "The doctor said that Gretchen doesn't have a diagnosis of osteoporosis, so we aren't treating her for that condition."

Isabel was exasperated by this erroneous claim, and asked a nurse to go through Gretchen's records with her to see when the diagnosis and treatment had disappeared.

On one type of document, the diagnosis still showed up as recently as a few weeks earlier. On another type of record, it had disappeared about a year earlier, with no explanation, and the drug had stopped being prescribed, too.

Yet in the record just before that one, the doctor had written, "Continue with the current treatment" for osteoporosis.

Isabel said to the nurse, "If you told me, 'We retested her and found that the treatment has been so successful that she doesn't need to take the drug anymore,' or, 'Because she is 90 years old, we have concluded that the drug poses more risks to her than it's worth,' I'd be fine with it. But to tell me that she doesn't have osteoporosis when you've been treating her for it for years—that's not right."

It turned out that the omission was due to a simple clerical error.

Isabel also found in her mother's file a consultation report from the endocrinologist who had been keeping an eye on Gretchen's thyroid nodules.

These growths are common and typically don't need to be treated. The doctor's report said that everything was okay and advised that Gretchen have another check-up in twelve months.

Isabel found herself nodding as she read. She had discussed this annual check-up in her mother's quarterly care planning conferences, in which she participated by phone.

All the key people and departments involved in Gretchen's care were part of those planning meetings, which are required by the federal government for people on Medicare. Everyone agreed that Gretchen would continue to get those annual check-ups.

Then she looked at the date on the consultation report. It was eighteen months earlier. Was the paperwork from a more recent visit misfiled? Or had the annual check-up not happened?

If Gretchen hadn't been taken to the doctor, was that the result of a deliberate change to the care plan that they had neglected to tell Isabel about? Or had they just forgotten to make the appointment?

A few hours after she asked, she was told, "Your mom is scheduled for the first available appointment with the endocrinologist, in about four weeks." They had simply neglected to make the appointment.

Isabel would have understood if the doctor had decided not to send her mother to the endocrinologist for some good reason.

For example, maybe there wasn't any treatment that could safely be given to someone Gretchen's age and in her condition. In that case, perhaps there was little point to getting the check-up.

But then a note in her chart should have explained this change. The chart is expected to include an accurate description of the individual's care plan.

It is not enough for the staff to say, "Oh, everyone knows she doesn't really need that."

The medical staff needs to document in the chart the reasoning for such a conclusion, or the resident's representative needs to have asked that the care not be given, in which case that fact needs to be documented as well.

In some cases, the staff may suggest that care wasn't given because the resident declined it. This can be a perfectly valid reason if the resident is mentally able to understand the pros and cons of the treatment and make a reasoned decision.

However, when a resident lacks the capacity to make reasoned choices, then any such decision to omit care would need to come from her representative.

35

Notice Obstacles That Impede Care

You may assume that your loved one is getting all the expected care in assisted living or nursing/skilled nursing. But sometimes, quirky problems disrupt the established routines in the facility, and care can suffer as a result.

Isabel turned to the section on dental care in her mother Gretchen's chart in the skilled nursing facility where Gretchen had been living for many years.

Isabel had agreed with the in-house dentist's recommendation that Gretchen have a check-up and get her teeth cleaned every three months. Gretchen had difficulty taking proper care of her teeth, but with the three-month check-ups, she had been doing well.

But Isabel was puzzled by the consultation request— the "work order" for a visit to the dentist. It showed that her mother was to have seen the dentist four months earlier, but it looked as if the appointment hadn't happened. The appointment request had two handwritten notes on it: "Refused!" and "Try 1x more."

Isabel asked the day nurse, "What does it mean when it says 'refused' on this dental visit order? Did my mother refuse to open her mouth so that the dentist could work on her teeth?"

"Oh, no," the nurse replied. "Your mother sometimes refuses to get in the elevator. We don't know why. That note probably means that that was a day that she wouldn't get in the elevator."

The in-house dentist was located one floor down. Because the building was built on a hill, the nursing wing where Gretchen lived was on a floor with direct access to the outside, and the dentist's office, even though it was a floor below, also was on a floor with an outside entrance.

Isabel and the nurse discussed the fact that at the extreme, someone could always put Gretchen in a car and drive her around to the entrance near the dentist's office.

But clearly, no one had thought to do that. They planned to take her on the elevator; when that didn't work, they didn't have a Plan B.

"Why does it say, 'Try 1x more' on here?" Isabel continued. "What does that mean—that if she refused to get on the elevator one more time, she would never get any more dental care for the rest of her life? That doesn't make any sense!"

The nurse sighed. "Yes, you're right." Isabel could picture the scene. The aide who had accompanied her mother would have come back in and reported, "Gretchen won't get on the elevator." A busy nurse would have said vaguely, "Okay, we'll try another time," before turning away to deal with another little crisis.

"But," Isabel said, "It doesn't look like another appointment was ever scheduled. It's been four months!"

When the unit secretary called to make a replacement appointment, she found that the lead-time was two months. So it would be nine months between appointments when it was supposed to be three. And if Isabel hadn't spoken up, no one would have ever rescheduled.

She frowned. Something else had just occurred to her. In the monthly bills she got from the nursing facility, there were always four or five charges for weekly appointments at the in-house hair salon—which was located on the bottom floor, just down the hall from the dentist.

Why were they able to take Gretchen downstairs to the hairdresser without fail—but unable to get her downstairs for health care appointments?

None of it made any sense!

A senior executive at the facility made an unexpectedly candid admission: "You know, no one actually reads the charts. They don't have time. They're too busy taking care of patients."

The nurses, she explained, get their information about what's happening in "Report," the meeting between shifts, when the departing nurses explain to the arriving nurses what has happened in the last eight to twelve hours and what they have to watch out for as a result.

A missed dental appointment wouldn't have made any impression at all.

The next several columns will discuss some approaches to take to find out what is happening with the care of your friend or relative, and how to address gaps and problems that you discover.

36

Read the Resident's Medical Chart

The last several articles in this series described some of the sorts of problems that can arise in even well run assisted living or skilled nursing facilities.

How can you tell if your friends or relatives are experiencing errors or oversights in their care?

A good first step is to read their medical charts. To do that, you need legal authorization.

A lawyer should draw up the document(s). Ideally, your loved one took this step long before moving into assisted living or skilled nursing. Once the facility has the document(s), you can ask to read the resident's chart.

Arizona law says that an assisted living resident's record must be "available for review by the resident or the [resident's] representative during normal business hours or at a time agreed upon by the resident and the manager."

A nursing home resident's medical records must be available for review "within one business day of the resident or the resident's representative's request," and you may obtain a copy to keep within two business days, although you might have to pay for the copying.

Be prepared for some nervousness on the part of the management, and be unfailingly cordial. They tend to assume that anyone who asks to see medical records intends to sue.

You may be able to reduce the tension by saying something like, "As my mother's health care representative, I feel a responsibility to understand her medical records so that I can ask intelligent questions and make informed decisions."

The first time you read your friend's or relative's medical record, ask that a staff member give you a tour of the document, which may be a three-ring binder with dozens of tabs. If the document is on a computer, the same request is relevant.

The chart will typically contain some basic information about the resident; an advance directive and/or living will; a DNR (Do Not Resuscitate) order if the individual or representative has signed one; a list of medicines and the doses that the resident is taking; doctors' notes from periodic (often monthly) exams; nurses' notes; summaries of any specialists' consultations; notes from other professionals or departments, such as a social worker, a dietician and an activities coordinator; medical test results; summaries of any physical therapy or other treatment;

summaries of quarterly care planning conferences attended by representatives of all key areas providing services to the resident; any doctors' orders not included in another section; and so forth.

One section of the chart in nursing homes is typically labeled MDS.

It includes a very lengthy and detailed document called the Minimum Data Set, which is generally required by Medicare even though Medicare typically doesn't pay for long-term care (nursing/skilled nursing) except for a short period under very limited circumstances.

It covers an extremely extensive array of topics such as hearing, vision, comprehension, mental acuity, memory, mood, behavior, preferences for daily routines and activities, ability to bathe, dress, use the toilet, eat, walk, control bowels and bladder, etc.

It also reports information about any and all diseases or conditions including pain; any recent falls; broken bones; any difficulty swallowing; percent of the typical meal actually eaten; condition of teeth; skin conditions including bed sores; medicines and other treatments; etc.

Once you know what sorts of information can be found in the chart, steps to take include:

1. Understand that you must not, under any circumstances, either write in the chart or remove anything. Have a pen and paper for taking notes, and sticky notes for flagging pages you have questions about.

2. Read the chart from front to back.

3. Take notes about anything that surprises or concerns you, that seems incorrect based on your knowledge of the resident, that is illegible, or that seems to conflict with the information on a different page. Jot down where the information appears so that you can find it again.

4. Ask the person helping you with the chart to explain any of these surprises or discrepancies.

5. If they cannot answer your questions on the spot, make note of any follow-ups agreed to, including when you will hear back and from whom.

37

Take Part In
Quarterly Care Planning Conferences

Many people are involved in caring for your friend or relative in a skilled nursing or nursing facility (long-term care): doctors, nurses, aides, dieticians, activities staff, social workers, possibly physical and occupational therapists, perhaps companions who don't perform medical services, and so forth.

How can you get attention to questions, concerns, or suggestions you have when a topic may involve several different departments?

If you have a topic that you want to discuss promptly, ask to speak to the person in charge of your loved one's care right away. Otherwise, take advantage of quarterly care planning conferences.

The federal government requires that these take place for all residents in long-term care facilities that are Medicare or Medicaid certified. As the name implies, they are scheduled every three months.

Tell the person in charge of your loved one's care— and the unit's secretary/clerk/administrative assistant— that you want to participate in these conferences.

They should then give you a couple weeks' notice of the date and time each quarter. If you cannot attend in person, ask that arrangements be made so that you can participate by calling in.

They will try to accommodate you by changing the schedule if you ask them to and if they can. However, because they are legally required to conduct the conferences at specific intervals, they can't delay the conference for three weeks because you are traveling, for instance.

They may not be able to change the day of the week, either, since they have to gather many people together who are already planning on participating in care planning conferences on the same day and time each week, such as Wednesday mornings from 9 a.m. to noon.

However, they may be able to make other changes, such as moving the conference up a week, or changing the time slot from 9 to 11 a.m.

Keep track of topics you would like to cover, and a week ahead of time, send the person in charge of your friend/relative's care an email explaining any issues you want to discuss in the conference. It helps to be specific.

For example, rather than writing, "How is she doing? Does she like the food?" you might say, "My mother's clothes seem loose on her. What is her weight now compared to three months ago? Are any dietary changes needed to help her maintain her weight?"

If you don't give the staff advance warning of the topics you want to discuss, often you will be told, "We'll check on that and get back to you."

This answer may not be very useful, for two reasons. First, based on my personal experience, such follow-ups can easily slip through the cracks. Second, you miss the chance to have several different departments participate with you in a discussion about how to address any issues.

If you think that the discussion you want to have will take a little while, ask that the meeting be scheduled for 30 minutes instead of the 15 minutes that they may routinely plan.

Typically, the staff will address any specifics you have raised, and each staff member will report on your friend/relative from their perspective.

For example, the person in charge of activities might say, "She really loves going on our bus every Sunday to local parks to see what's blooming, and she loves any music programs we offer. We've started a little photography group; we lend the residents digital cameras to use, and she took some really great pictures of the stream and the irises in the park last week."

The nutritionist might say, "We've started giving her a Magic Cup (nutritionally fortified ice cream) at dinner every night because she's only eating about half her meal but she'll always eat the ice cream. Her BMI (body mass index) is in the low-normal range, so we don't want her to lose any more weight. We'll start adding Med Pass (a nutrition shake) at lunch if she is still losing weight in a month."

Despite this chance to share information, it's still important to read your loved one's chart to identify any gaps or discrepancies that might not surface in care planning conferences.

38

Take Additional Steps To Learn About a Loved One's Care

Previous articles mentioned that you can read your loved one's medical chart and participate in care planning conferences. This article offers additional suggestions about how you might get—and keep—yourself in the loop.

Find out what records and care plans for your relative do not appear in her chart. A knowledgeable member of staff (typically a nurse) should be able to tell you.

For example, it is customary to weigh residents once a month. It is easier for the staff to record weights for 30 people on one piece of paper, rather than haul 30 resident's three-ring binders down the hall to the scale area and record the weights in those 30 different binders.

As a result, they may have a notebook that has one page per month and lists everyone's weight on that page.

As another example, aides typically care for several residents. They may have care instructions for all the people they take care of printed out on one piece of paper, instead of having a separate page for each resident. That's more convenient for them, and saves on printing costs.

But those instructions won't appear in your relative's chart, because they include information about other people.

Thus, it's useful to ask what records are grouped by record type (e.g., weight) or staff member or shift (e.g., care instructions), and ask how you can get copies of those records as they pertain to your relative.

If anything in those records seems out of place, ask the staff to confirm that they are the notes for your loved one.

Because the records are grouped by record type instead of by resident, it is easy for a mistake to be made and for you to be told information that belongs to a resident other than the one you are asking about.

Read the resident's contract with the facility. This should be available when the resident moves in; at times, it might not be available for about two weeks. Look for care that is described as excluded from the contract.

You might think that the daily or monthly fee would cover all routine medical care for a resident in a nursing facility (long-term care). But that's often not the case.

For example, the contract for one continuing care community (which offers all levels of care from independent living to skilled nursing) notes that the resident must pay for refractions done during eye exams, glasses or contact lenses, podiatry (foot care), hearing tests and hearing aids, dental care, psychiatric care, treatment for addictions, dialysis, most durable medical equipment, and anything that Medicare won't cover.

Faced with such a list, it would be reasonable for you to ask how arrangements are made for periodic eye exams, new glasses, dental care, and so forth.

Because these fall outside the scope of the facility's responsibilities, arranging for these items may easily fall through the cracks, so it is important to agree on what care is needed and then check to make sure that the care is being delivered as intended.

Ask if the facility has a family council. This is a group of family members of residents who get together periodically to share experiences, learn from each other, and get support for the difficult task of being the responsible party for a family member who is no longer able to handle her own affairs.

If a council exists, attend at least one or two meetings to see if you can learn from others' experiences. For example, other residents' family members may have learned about staffing or program changes that you didn't know about. They may know who to call to solve a type of problem you haven't been able to get resolved.

If such a council doesn't exist and the idea interests you, one option is to propose that one be created, understanding that you might be asked to lead it.

Get to know the people involved in caring for, or making decisions about, your relative. Keep track of their names. Get their business cards or at least try to get their work phone numbers and email addresses.

A great deal of information about residents is communicated among staff members orally, so sometimes the only way to find out what has been happening with your loved one is to talk with the staff.

Over time, you may find that you build up quite a contact list, including people in roles such as medical director, director of nursing, director of health services, assisted living or skilled nursing unit manager, doctors, nurses, charge nurse, floor nurse, certified nursing assistants, licensed vocational nurses, aides, companions, social worker, records manager, fitness manager, physical therapy manager, dietician, therapeutic recreation (activities) manager, accounts receivable manager, insurance billing manager, unit secretary, on-site dentist, on-site hair stylist, and so forth.

Next week's column will discuss what to do if you run into roadblocks.

39

Get Help
If Problems Persist

If you feel that the care your relative is receiving in assisted living or another long-term care setting isn't acceptable, what can you do? First, talk with a nurse or the individual identified as responsible for your loved one's care.

If you aren't satisfied with the results of that conversation, speak with the individual in charge of the assisted living or long-term care unit.

It almost always works best to remain polite and cordial. Explain the gap you have observed, for example, "My aunt is supposed to be getting food that is very easy to chew. But the last two times I visited, I saw food on her tray such as a chicken breast, an apple, and a hard roll. She didn't eat any of them. She has lost weight."

Then explain the change you are asking for. You might say, for example, "How can we ensure that she is served food she can chew at every meal, starting with the next meal?"

Often, issues can be resolved immediately. Most facilities are staffed with people who genuinely want to do the right thing.

If issues persist, you might send a cordial letter to the person in charge of the unit, documenting your concerns and efforts to get resolution, including specific details, dates, times, and employees' names if known.

Explain the result you are looking for and ask what changes will be made to achieve it and when. Ask for a reply by a specific date, based on the urgency of the issue.

To learn what it is reasonable to expect of care facilities, consider crawling through the requirements detailed in state regulations. While not light reading, the law typically covers everything from the minimum size for a bedroom to how far ahead menus should be posted. To see the requirements spelled out in Arizona state law, go to http://www.azsos.gov/public_services/Title_09/9-10.htm.

Article 7 addresses assisted living, and Article 9 covers nursing facilities (nursing/skilled nursing/long-term care). Clicking on the title of an Article calls up its detail. Ignore all the legalese about the history of the section and enactment of the rules.

Assisted living facilities are required to provide a copy of residents' rights when an individual is admitted, along with phone numbers for the Arizona Department of

Health Services' Office of Assisted Living Licensure, which sets standards for assisted living, performs inspections, and investigates complaints; Arizona Adult Protective Services, which investigates claims of abuse, neglect, or exploitation; Arizona Long-Term Care Ombudsman, which can help residents and families understand their rights and help address complaints; and several other agencies.

Nursing units (long-term care facilities) are required to post information about their license and their quality rating from the Arizona Department of Health Services, as well as contact information for the Department's Office of Long-Term Care Licensing, which licenses, inspects, and investigates complaints about such facilities; and the state's Long-Term Care Ombudsman and Adult Protective Services, which address issues in long-term care as well as in assisted living as noted above.

Facilities are required to have written procedures for addressing resident complaints, and they are not permitted to retaliate when complaints are raised.

What if you are in independent living, so all those health care rules don't apply, but you are age 60 or older and feel that you are being mistreated by your landlord?

The Elder Rights Program, run by the Area Agency on Aging of the Northern Arizona Council of Governments, may be able to help.

They give first priority to low-income and otherwise disadvantaged seniors, and can help address landlord-tenant disputes and other housing issues.

They can also help with legal documents such as living wills and with government benefit programs such as Social Security.

The Legal Advocacy Program can be reached at (928) 775-9993 x4271, or you may search online for Northern Arizona Elder Rights Program.

What's the bottom line? If something is going wrong with your or a relative's senior housing, or with care in an assisted living or nursing/skilled nursing facility, you don't have to suffer in silence.

Many, many protections are built into the law, and many helping hands are willing to assist you if problems remain unresolved. You don't have to put up with substandard conditions or care.

VIII

The Future
of Retirement Care

A new approach to caring for the elderly has surfaced within the last decade. It can help make it more likely that the last years of life will be satisfying and meaningful.

40

The Green House Movement

What do you think of when you hear the term "green house?" A glass building designed to house tender plants? A home that is a model of energy efficiency, perhaps producing as much power as it uses?

Get ready for a third meaning. The Green House Project (www.greenhouseproject.org) is an approach to designing, staffing, and running an assisted living or nursing/skilled nursing facility to make the residents the true focus and center of attention.

It is designed specifically to encourage and support ongoing growth and development in even its oldest residents.

What distinguishes a Green House from a typical assisted living or long-term care facility? A Green House video explains, "The goal is a complete transformation. . .

from an institutional setting. . . that when you or I walk into it, we think, 'Please don't ever let me have to live here,'—into something warm. . . that you or I would walk into and think, 'I'd be happy living here, or I would be happy to have somebody I really cared about living here.'"

The buildings are deliberately designed to be homelike for 10-12 residents, offering each resident a private room with its own full bathroom.

In contrast, nursing/skilled nursing facilities usually offer only a half-bath in the room, with showers typically taken in a large, impersonal shower room.

The private rooms open off a common area that includes a living room, an open kitchen, and a dining area with one large table—a sort of outsized version of a standard home with an open floor plan.

The vast majority of the care that residents receive is provided by caregivers called Shabazim, who as a team manage the home. They cook, clean, and do laundry in addition to providing hands-on care for the residents.

Because meals are prepared in a large kitchen that is right out in the open, residents can see and hear and smell the meals as they are made.

They are welcome to talk with whoever is cooking and may even help out in the kitchen if they want. In contrast, meals in traditional care facilities arrive from behind closed doors, prepared by professionals who the residents rarely see or interact with.

In a Green House, staff members sit and eat at the large dining table interspersed with the residents. They all share the same food, and they all engage in the conversation around the table.

Of course, the staff will help residents who need assistance eating; the general impression, though, is that the residents and staff are all part of one large family.

The residents spend their time on a variety of activities that have meaning for them individually. A staff member and a resident may spend hours talking, and it is common for them to develop very close bonds.

Bill Thomas, the founder of the movement, noted in a video interview, "Here's the problem. . . conventional long-term care makes the doctors and nurses the star of the show. And so they are out in front, they're in the spotlight 100 percent of the time. The Green House makes the elders stars of the show. They're the ones in the spotlight. And the nurses and doctors are still there, but they're backstage, where they ought to be."

The Green House model is supported by a well-run national program that offers extensive practical support in the areas of building architecture and design, financial analysis related to creating and running Green Houses, regulatory compliance, leadership training and employee development.

In Arizona, Green House homes can be found in the Phoenix area. See a video about Green House projects at http://thegreenhouseproject.org/green-house-model.

In summary, the Green House model presents hope for the future of elder care, because it finds ways to honor and respect elderly residents for who they are, rather than acting as if the most important fact about them is that they have some malfunctioning body parts.

ABOUT THE AUTHOR

Elizabeth L. Bewley writes a weekly newspaper column called "The Good Patient" for the Prescott, Arizona *Daily Courier*. She earns high praise for making complex topics easy to understand.

Bewley analyzes pitfalls that await the unsuspecting when they interact with the health care system in any of its many forms and locations—and describes easy action steps anyone can take to sidestep problems and get better care.

She founded Pario Health Institute in 2008 after 20 years as an executive with health care icon Johnson & Johnson. Her goal is to drive change so that the purpose of health care becomes *to enable people to lead the lives they want*.

Bewley earned an MBA from Columba and is a certified Six Sigma Black Belt with extensive experience in fixing broken processes to get significantly better results.

Her unwavering advocacy for people using the health care system is informed by her own near-death experiences— including one resulting from a bicycle crash at 44 mph.

She lives in Prescott, AZ with her husband Stephen R. Brubaker, and enjoys hiking and mountain biking in the surrounding area.

See www.pariohealth.net and www.killercure.net for more information about Bewley's work and publications.